P9-BZM-624

Research in
Social Group Work

The *Social Work with Groups* series

Series Editors: Catherine P. Papell and Beulah Rothman

- *Co-Leadership in Social Work with Groups*, Catherine P. Papell and Beulah Rothman

- *Social Groupwork & Alcoholism*, Marjorie Altman and Ruth Crocker, Guest Editors

- *Groupwork with the Frail Elderly*, Shura Saul, Guest Editor

- *The Use of Group Services in Permanency Planning for Children*, Sylvia Morris, Guest Editor

- *Activities and Action in Groupwork*, Ruth Middleman, Guest Editor

- *Groupwork with Women/Groupwork with Men: An Overview of Gender Issues in Social Groupwork Practice*, Beth Glover Reed and Charles D. Garvin, Guest Editors

- *Ethnicity in Social Group Work Practice*, Larry Davis, Guest Editor

- *Time as a Factor in Groupwork*, Albert Alissi and Max Casper, Guest Editors

- *Groupwork with Children and Adolescents*, Ralph Kolodny and James Garland, Guest Editors

- *The Legacy of William Schwartz: Group Practice as Shared Interaction*, Alex Gitterman and Lawrence Shulman, Guest Editors

- *Research in Social Group Work*, Sheldon D. Rose and Ronald A. Feldman, Guest Editors

- *Collectivity in Social Group Work: Concept and Practice* (forthcoming), Norma C. Lang and Joanne Sulman, Guest Editors

Research in
Social Group Work

Sheldon D. Rose and Ronald A. Feldman
Editors

The Haworth Press
New York • London

Research in Social Group Work has also been published as *Social Work with Groups*, Volume 9, Number 3, Fall 1986.

The Haworth Press, Inc., 12 West 32 Street, New York, NY 10001
EUROSPAN/Haworth, 3 Henrietta Street, London, WC2E 8LU England

Library of Congress Cataloging-in-Publication Data

Research in social group work.

Includes bibliographies.
1. Social group work. 2. Small groups. I. Rose, Sheldon D.
II. Feldman, Ronald A.
HV45.R47   1987   361.4   86-29526
ISBN 0-86656-645-7

Research in Social Group Work

Social Work with Groups
Volume 9, Number 3

CONTENTS

Research in
Social Group Work

EDITORIAL

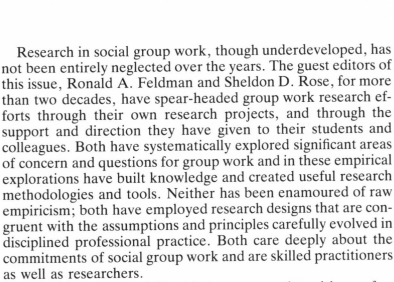

Research in social group work, though underdeveloped, has not been entirely neglected over the years. The guest editors of this issue, Ronald A. Feldman and Sheldon D. Rose, for more than two decades, have spear-headed group work research efforts through their own research projects, and through the support and direction they have given to their students and colleagues. Both have systematically explored significant areas of concern and questions for group work and in these empirical explorations have built knowledge and created useful research methodologies and tools. Neither has been enamoured of raw empiricism; both have employed research designs that are congruent with the assumptions and principles carefully evolved in disciplined professional practice. Both care deeply about the commitments of social group work and are skilled practitioners as well as researchers.

The articles selected for this issue are authored by professionals who are motivated by the desire to improve and extend knowledge. Each paper represents activity of curious minds at work with purposeful direction. Thus this special issue of *Social Work with Groups* can add to the growing base from which contemporary and future group work research can be built. It signifies a new stage of maturity in the assessment and validation of our practice.

CP
BR

GUEST EDITORIAL

As noted in the lead article of this special research issue of *Social Work with Groups,* research in social group work is on the increase. Yet, even so, both the quantity and the quality of the current research are insufficient to assure that group work practice will be based firmly upon systematic scientific research. The present issue of this journal represents an effort to take stock of group work research and to advance the research base of the field even if only in very modest terms. The articles that appear in the issue reflect not only advances and strengths in group work research but also some of the deficiencies and gaps that characterize contemporary research in the field.

Special thanks for preparation of this issue are in order for four group work scholars who assisted us in an editorial capacity: Larry Davis, Washington University, St. Louis; Maeda Galinsky, University of North Carolina; Martin Sundel, University of Texas at Arlington, and James K. Whittaker, University of Washington. It should be noted that only three of the articles that appear here were prepared expressly for the present issue, namely, those by Anderson, Feldman, and Goldberg and Lamont. The others emerged from the first meeting in June 1985 of the Symposium on the Empirical Foundations of Group Work. This symposium represents in its own right a timely and promising mechanism for advancing the scientific knowledge base of social group work.

The symposium was planned in the lobbies of the hotels in which the annual conferences of the Committee for the Advancement of Social Work with Groups, and the Association for the Advancement of Behavior Therapy were held. The former conference appeared to provide too limited a forum for the exchange of research and methodological advances since it was confined solely to group work, while the latter was deficient in attending to theory, empirical findings, and methodological issues that concern practice within the profession. The originators of the symposium sought to develop a forum in which the formal and informal exchange of research ideas and procedures could be applied to a wide variety of groups.

Although lightly attended, this first research symposium was considered a success by the participants. All sections of the country were represented. The limited size of the symposium made it possible to discuss the formal presentations at length and to examine the many problems that are inherent in the evaluation of progress and outcome in group work. As is evident by the contents of the present issue, many of the papers were of publishable quality. They focused both upon methodological problems and current research. A welcome outcome of the symposium was a decision to plan a second meeting for Ann Arbor, Michigan on June 17–19th, 1986, with a theme of Process and Outcome.

The articles that are presented here attend to many different facets of group work research. Thus, for example, Feldman documents trends and deficits in group work research over the past two decades. Glisson examines a key methodological issue in group work research by discussing the discrepancies that may exist between analyses which incorporate the individual as the unit of analysis and those which employ the group as the key unit of analysis. To help scholars delineate fruitful areas for future research, Tallant discusses how meta-analyses of clusters of group work studies can be performed.

Garvin demonstrates the complexities and many of the problems that confront group work researchers by describing the features of an emerging study of task-centered group work with chronic mental patients. In a similar vein, Subramanian reviews a study of group training for the management of chronic pain in interpersonal situations. Rose, Tallant, Tolman and Subramanian then present a comprehensive discussion of program development research in the multimethod group approach. Goldberg and Lamont, in the next article, review the findings of a study which suggests that a group work curriculum exerts a discernible differential impact on the learning of social work students. And, finally, Anderson addresses one of the fundamental and enduring issues in social group work, namely, the integration between research and practice.

In short, the articles in this special issue address a broad range of critical concerns in group work research. Even further, they report initial, albeit sometimes rudimentary, efforts to advance the research knowledge base of social group work. It is our hope and expectation that this issue represents the first of a series of special research issues of *Social Work with Groups*. Such collections will not merely reflect research progress in the field; more important, they will promote and stimulate crucial advances in group work research. Their value will be inestimable because systematic, sustained and rigorous research still represents the key to comprehending and resolving the many theoretical, methodological, and practice problems that inhere in social group work.

Sheldon D. Rose
Ronald A. Feldman

Group Work Knowledge
and Research:
A Two-Decade Comparison

Ronald A. Feldman

The last major survey of the knowledge base of social group work was published two decades ago. Following an extensive review of social group work articles published during an eight-year period, Marvin Silverman (1966) concluded that there were serious shortcomings in the available literature. Of particular interest with reference to the present issue of *Social Work with Groups,* he found that group work articles regarding applications of social science, innovations in practice theory, and research and surveys constituted only 15% of the reviewed literature. Instead, the majority of the literature offered descriptions of specific programs or areas of group work practice. As Silverman noted, the former types of articles are aimed at expanding the scientific knowledge base of social group work. Yet, in view of their paucity, he concluded that the need for scientific knowledge development in social group work had been amply demonstrated by his study. Not surprisingly, perhaps, 8% of the articles that were surveyed in his study constituted appeals for knowledge or for more rigorous scientific research. Silverman noted accordingly that "one would hope that in the future more authors will heed their own advice—carry out research and build theory—rather than plead for others to do it" (p. 58).

The present review is designed to ascertain how, if at all,

Ronald A. Feldman is Professor and Associate Dean, Columbia University School of Social Work, New York, New York, and Director, Center for Adolescent Mental Health, George Warren Brown School of Social Work, Washington University, St. Louis, Missouri.

Appreciation is expressed to Virginia Fagersberg, Anita Martin and Barbara Zawin for assistance in literature review and classification.

the knowledge base of social group work has changed during the two decades since publication of Silverman's landmark article. During this period doctoral programs in social work proliferated greatly. New research journals were launched by the profession and, of more direct import, journals that focus expressly upon social group work were established. Consequently, one might expect major changes in the knowledge base of social group work during this period. The presumption, of course, is that the current knowledge base would be considerably more scientific with respect to its grounding in research and the systematic application of social science principles. To investigate this assumption and related ones, the present manuscript reports a replication of Silverman's study for a recent eight-year period. The same classification categories are employed in both studies.

METHOD

The study performed by Silverman is based upon a review of all social group work articles contained in the periodicals *Social Work* and *Social Service Review* throughout the 1956–1964 period. In addition, Silverman reviewed group work articles that appeared in edited collections prepared under the aegis of the National Association of Social Workers and the National Conference on Social Welfare. In particular, these are: *Group Work and Community Organization, 1956; Group Work Papers, 1957; Social Work with Groups, 1958, 1959,* and *1960; New Perspectives on Services to Groups;* and *Social Work Practice, 1962, 1963,* and *1964* (for full citations, see Silverman, 1966:56).

The present study likewise examines the periodicals *Social Work* and *Social Service Review* for an eight-year period (1975 through 1983). In addition, it concludes the following journals for the same time period: *Clinical Social Work Journal; Social Service Research; Social Work Research and Abstracts;* and *Sociology and Social Welfare.* The present study also surveyed publications in *Social Work with Groups* from 1978 (when the journal was established) through 1983 and in *Practice Digest* from 1980 (when this journal was established) through 1983. Only 18 issues of the above-cited journals were not available for review and, therefore, for inclusion in the study. The present study does not include any of the edited collections that were surveyed by Silverman; all had ceased publication since the time of his study. Both studies are conspicuous by virtue of their exclusion of group work texts. Furthermore, the 1986 study does not include articles from *Behavior Group Therapy.* Hence, it somewhat underestimates the amount of group work research in recent years.

In both the 1966 study and the 1986 study, each reviewed article was classified into one of eleven categories. These are described succinctly as follows:

1. *Descriptions.* These articles describe specific programs, agency services, or particular groups. They are predominantly concrete. Citations from recordings are frequent.
2. *Areas of practice.* Articles in this category discuss a specific area of practice such as group work in medical settings, supervision, work with delinquent gangs, and use of volunteers. As Silverman notes, they are to be distinguished from Category 7, "innovations in practice theory," because no organized attempt is made to reconceptualize traditional practice theory.
3. *Appeals for knowledge.* Articles in this category stress the need for expanding and systematizing the knowledge base of social group work. Included are appeals for research, integration of social science material, and the development of practice theory. Some articles are fashioned in highly general terms while others suggest specific guidelines and approaches.
4. *Appeals for direction of service.* These articles aim to persuade group workers to place greater or lesser emphasis on specific programs or certain areas of service. Some articles are based upon extensive rationales or citations of the available literature while others are based primarily on ethical arguments.
5. *Traditional statements of principles.* Articles in this category are a mixture of broadly conceived practice principles and rather general ethical prescriptions. For the most part, they are restatements of the traditional conceptual and value base of the field.

6. *Applications of social science.* These articles attempt to utilize theories, concepts, or research findings from the social sciences and apply them to some aspect of social group work.
7. *Innovations in practice theory.* Articles in this category deal with the establishment of a framework which selectively guides the activity of the worker. As noted by Silverman, they are to be distinguished from Category 5 in that an attempt is made to reformulate practice theory.
8. *Research and surveys.* These articles seek to make a contribution to knowledge through the empirical testing of hypotheses or the compilation of facts in a specified area.
9. *Group work-casework-group therapy relationships.* Articles in this category typically compare group work with more "clinical" orientations. Some also describe a particular program in which group workers and caseworkers collaborate with one another.
10. *Historical articles.* These articles present social group work or some aspect of it in historical perspective.
11. *Social group work education.* Articles in this category focus directly upon graduate education in social group work.

The vast majority of articles reviewed for both the 1966 study and the 1986 study were assigned readily to one of these eleven categories. Whenever an article could fit into more than a single category, however, assignment was based on its *primary* emphasis. Hence, the 1966 and 1986 studies are identical in terms of the categories and criteria employed for the classification of articles.

FINDINGS

The comparative data for the two study periods are reported in Table 1. The most visible finding pertains to the marked growth in the *volume* of group work literature during the 1975–1983 period. Thus, the total number of group work articles nearly tripled from 106 in the 1956–1964 period to 302

Table 1 : CLASSIFICATION OF SELECTED ARTICLES, 1966 vs. 1986

CATEGORY	NUMBER		PERCENTAGE	
	1966	1986	1966	1986
1. Descriptions	32	146	30	48
2. Areas of practice	27	34	25	11
3. Appeals for knowledge	9	2	8	1
4. Appeals for direction of service	7	12	7	4
5. Traditional statements of principles	8	26	8	9
6. Applications of social science	7	16	7	5
7. Innovations in practice theory	4	16	4	5
8. Research and surveys	4	29	4	10
9. Group work-casework-group therapy relationships	5	6	5	2
10. Historical articles	2	3	2	1
11. Social group work education	1	12	1	4
	106	302	101*	100

* Percentage is greater than 100% due to rounding error.

in the 1975–1983 period. In part, of course, this finding is a reflection of the larger number of journals surveyed in the latter study. Yet, it also reflects the emergence of new journals that have promoted group work publication during the last two decades. For instance, *Social Work with Groups, Practice Digest, Social Service Research, Social Work Research and Abstracts, Sociology and Social Welfare, Clinical Social Work Journal,* and *Behavior Group Therapy* were not even in existence at the time of the 1966 study. In fact, articles in *Social Work with Groups*—the only one of the cited journals that focuses expressly upon group work—account for 55% of the total articles reviewed for the 1986 study.

The present study seeks to examine changes not only in the volume of group work literature but, more important, variations in the *types* of publications that have appeared. With particular reference to the present issue of *Social Work with Groups,* the most pronounced change in the last two decades pertains to articles regarding group work research. Research articles and surveys more than doubled during this period from 4% to 10% of the reviewed literature. Nevertheless, it can be argued that the latter figure reflects far too little research for a field of practice that hopes to be based upon scientific knowledge. This observation is all the more trenchant when one considers not only the quantity of the available research but its quality as well. Indeed, very few of the 29 studies reviewed for the 1986 article are characterized by the application of statistical tests or, even, by control groups, baseline periods, or the analysis of more than a score of subjects.

Articles concerning group work education also increased in number over the past two decades. They constituted 4% of the literature in the 1986 study but only 1% in the 1966 study. Even so, such articles represent a very small portion of the available literature. Likewise, historical articles constituted a negligible portion of the literature both in the 1986 study (1%) and the 1966 study (2%). In the 1986 study (2%) there also were fewer articles that compared group work, casework, and group therapy than in the 1966 study (5%). Furthermore, the 1986 study revealed fewer appeals for knowledge than the 1966 study (respectively, 1% vs. 8%) and fewer appeals regarding the direction of service (respectively, 4% vs. 7%). Perhaps, then, group workers have now progressed beyond mere appeals and toward the articulation of substantive knowledge and guidelines for the direction of service.

Nevertheless, relatively similar portions of the literature in both studies represent mere restatements of traditional principles. Thus, in the 1986 study 9% of the literature represented traditional statements or restatements of practice principles and ethical prescriptions. This is roughly the same as two decades earlier (viz., 8%). Moreover, the application of social science principles decreased somewhat during the past two decades from 7% of the literature to 5%. Innovations in practice theory hardly varied at all during this period. In the 1966 study they constituted 4% of the group work literature while in 1986 they constituted 5% of the literature.

Perhaps the best indicator of the relatively unchanging nature of the group work literature inheres in the finding that in both 1966 and 1986 the preponderance of the reviewed literature consisted merely of descriptions of specific programs or particular areas of group work practice. These two categories constituted 55% of the literature in the 1966 study and 59% in the 1986 study. Within these categories, however, it is pertinent to note that program descriptions increased from 30% to 48% of the literature in two decades while articles regarding areas of practice declined from 25% to 11%. These findings may reflect the fact that it has become increasingly difficult over the years to delineate new substantive areas for the application of social group work. By contrast, it may be somewhat easier to discover new sites for group work practice or new ways to apply knowledge already in existence.

SUMMARY AND CONCLUSIONS

Comparison of the group work literature from two different periods of time (namely, 1956–1964 and 1975–1983) indicates a growing emphasis upon systematic research. Nevertheless, both the quantity and the quality of the extant research are inadequate for a profession that wishes its practice principles to be grounded in scientific study. Publications that pertain to "applications of social science," "innovations in practice theory," and "research and surveys" are aimed at expanding the scientific knowledge base of social group work. Together, these kinds of publications constitute a larger portion of the literature reviewed in 1986 (20%) than two decades earlier (15%). Overall, however, the increase is a rather modest one.

Substantive patterns in the recent group work literature and in the literature of two decades ago appear to be strikingly similar in most major respects. Relatively equal portions of both literatures are devoted to traditional statements of principles, applications of social science knowledge, innovations in practice theory, and historical articles. Likewise, both literatures consist predominantly of descriptions of specific programs and particular areas of group work practice. Somewhat fewer publications in the 1986 study are concerned about the similarities, differences, or interfaces among group work, casework, and group therapy. Conversely, a somewhat larger portion of the recent literature focuses upon group work education.

In contrast with the situation two decades ago, a smaller segment of the recent literature is devoted to appeals for knowledge or direction regarding group work service. This trend partially fulfills Silverman's hope "that in the future more authors will heed their own advice—carry out research and build theory—rather than plead for others to do it" (1966:58). Yet, given the rather scant amount of research reported in both studies, it is evident that such appeals still are very much in order. This is particularly so with reference to knowledge that is based upon systematic scientific study. In short, the research base of social group work is growing, but much remains to be done before group workers can safely claim that their practice is well-grounded in scientific research.

REFERENCE

Silverman, Marvin, "Knowledge in Social Group Work: A Review of the Literature," *Social Work*, 1966, *11*, 3, 56–62.

The Group versus the Individual as the Unit of Analysis in Small Group Research

Charles Glisson

ABSTRACT. It is common for social work researchers to use the individual as the unit of analysis in small group research. This paper examines the discrepancies that may exist between analyses that incorporate the individual and those that incorporate the group as the unit of analysis. An example is presented with data collected from 331 members of 53 workgroups in 22 different human service organizations. Researchers are cautioned against drawing conclusions about groups from data based on the individual as the unit of analysis.

THE PROBLEM

The question of the appropriate unit of analysis in social and behavioral science research has received little empirical or theoretical attention. This is because the behavior, attitude and affect of individuals have been the major foci of applied research efforts. It is only when the social scientist turns to collectives (collections of individuals) as phenomena of interest that the appropriate unit of analysis becomes an issue. In social work, over sixty-three percent of the research published in five major journals over a six year period incorporated the individual as the unit of analysis. The second most common unit of analysis was the organization (16%), followed by the family (5%), country (4.4%), small group (3.5%), state (3%), journal article or document (2.4%), and community or city (2%) (Glisson, 1983).

Charles Glisson is Professor, School of Social Work, University of Hawaii, Honolulu, Hawaii 96822.

15

Frequently, researchers who intend to study collectives utilize the individual rather than the collective as the unit of empirical analysis although the phenomena of interest are conceptualized at higher levels, i.e., family, small group, organization (examples from small group research are Schopler and Galinsky, 1981; Davis, 1979; Lawrence and Walter, 1978; Feldman and Caplinger, 1977). In fact, of the social work research published in the six year period mentioned above, less than half of the research concerning small group phenomena (27%) actually used the group as the unit of analysis (examples are Toseland, Rivas, and Chapman, 1984; Segal, 1982). Further, those researchers that do incorporate higher levels of analysis often aggregate the responses of individuals to obtain data that describe larger units such as families, groups, or organizations (examples are Rose, 1981; Glisson and Martin, 1980).

Table 1 provides a summary of the possible research strategies for studying small groups. As shown, it is possible to incorporate either the individual or the group as the unit of analysis in the four designs. As mentioned, most of the small group research published in social work journals uses the individual as the unit of analysis and, therefore, is distributed over the row labeled A. The research using either unit of analysis, moreover, is not equally distributed over the four designs. The most common design reported for social work small group research is the survey (57%), followed by idiographic (19%), and quasi-experimental and experiental (11% each) (Glisson, 1983).

The general question raised here concerns the differences between research strategies A and B, and the implications of those differences for small group research. Two specific issues will be addressed. The first issue concerns the appropriateness of using the individual as the unit of analysis in studying collectives such as small groups. The second issue concerns the implications of aggregating the responses of individuals (Strategy A) as a means of incorporating the collective (Strategy B) as the unit of analysis. The first issue rests on the theoretical conceptualization of the research question and the second issue involves the empirical implications of describing a collective by averaging the characteristics of its individual parts.

Table 1

Research Strategies for Studying Small Groups

Unit of Analysis	Design			
	1. Idiographic (N=1)	2. Survey	3. Quasi-experimental	4. Experimental
A. Individual	examine characteristics over time of one individual subjected to one or more group conditions	examine relationships among characteristics of individuals under one or more group conditions (The most common strategy in S.W. group research)	compare groups of nonrandomly assigned individuals under two or more conditions	compare groups of randomly assigned individuals under two or more conditions
B. Group	examine characteristics over time of one group under one or more conditions	examine relationships among characteristics of sample of groups	compare groups of nonrandomly assigned groups under two or more conditions	compare groups of randomly assigned groups under two or more conditions

17

THE INDIVIDUAL AS THE UNIT OF ANALYSIS
IN SMALL GROUP RESEARCH

As reported above, over half of the social work research concerning groups uses the individual as the unit of analysis. In other words, most of the published group research is explicitly focusing on individuals in an attempt to understand group phenomena.

An evaluation of this approach to studying groups requires a brief digression. All social science inquiry is prompted by the existence of variation. More accurately, perhaps, without variation social science would take on an entirely different form. We take this point for granted, because it is hard to imagine a social world without variation. In such a world, all individuals would share the same characteristics and all collectives would share the same characteristics in some Orwellian society of automatons. Nevertheless, it is the variation that most of us take for granted that social scientists specifically seek to understand. They seek to understand variation through the study of covariation. When variables covary, variation in one variable is "understood" by the concomitant variation in another variable.

When individuals are the units of analysis in small group research, variation and covariation are reported for variables that characterize individuals. In some group research using this approach, the individuals are members of a single group and in others, the individuals are distributed over more than one group. In the former case, analysis is restricted to the within-group variation of individuals and in the latter, is extended to include the between-group variation of individuals as well. In either case, it is the variation in individuals rather than the variation in groups that provides the data for conclusions. An example illustrates the importance of the distinction.

Figure 1 presents data for 36 individuals plotted on the two dimensional space defined by the variables X and Y. The individuals are distributed across three groups: A_1, A_2 and A_3. Notice that there is a rather strong positive relationship between X and Y for these 36 individuals. Also, there is a slight relationship between the nominal variable A, referring to group membership, and Y. A_1 has the highest Y values and

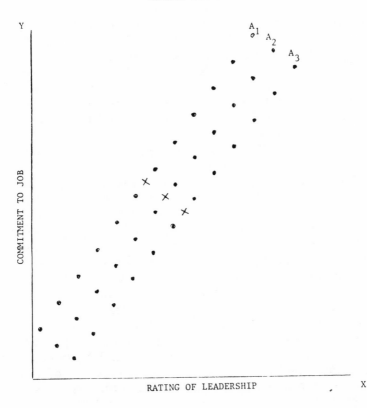

Stylized Distribution of Values for Individuals (N=36)

in Three Work Groups (A$_1$, A$_2$, A$_3$)

FIGURE 1

A$_3$ the lowest. The relationship between A and Y, however, is insignificant because the within-group variation is much greater than the between-group variation. A similar pattern exists between A and X.

If the unit of analysis was the group, however, only three

data points would be plotted. A_1, A_2, and A_3 would no longer represent values for the nominal variable, A, but would represent the three groups as the units of analysis. Depending on the nature of the variables, X and Y could be used to describe the three group units just as X and Y were used to describe the 36 units of individuals. A, however, as a variable, would have disappeared. The N = 36 study would be transformed into an N = 3 study.

The choice of the appropriate unit of analysis depends upon the research question and the theoretical model upon which it is based. If the question concerns covariation among variables that describe individuals, the appropriate unit is the individual. If the question concerns covariation among variables that describe groups, the appropriate unit is the group.

Confusion over the correct choice results from the failure to empirically distinguish between variables that describe characteristics of individuals and variables that describe characteristics of groups. In the above example, the N = 36 study incorporated a variable, A, that has three levels or values. These values describe characteristics of individuals, not of groups. Of course, there are certainly three groups that can be distinguished by the values of A_1, A_2, and A_3, but conceptually and empirically these are groupings of individuals formed by their sharing a characteristic, either A, A_2, or A_3. "A" could be an active factor manipulated by the research or an assigned factor that results from an inherent characteristic of each subject. The point here is that in this instance it is the covariation of variables that describe the individuals that would be assessed using the 36 subjects.

It is important to emphasize that conclusions could not be drawn from these data about the covariation among variables that characterize the groups. Conclusions, rather, would focus on the behavior, attitude, or affect of the individuals under certain group conditions (A_1, A_2, A_3).

As an example, imagine that Figure 1 represents a study of small work groups delivering mental health services. A_1, A_2, and A_3 represent three work groups. An objective of the research is to determine the relationship between how the head of each group performs as a leader (X) and the members' commitment to their jobs (Y). Other objectives are to determine if that relationship is homogeneous for the three groups and if there is a difference in commitment across the three groups. In other words, the study intends to examine the two possible main effects and the possible interaction effect of X and A on Y.

Figure 1 shows a strong relationship between leadership (X) and commitment (Y), an insignificant relationship between group (A) and commitment, and no interaction effect of X and A on Y. More accurately, it shows that *individuals* who rate their work group leader highly report more commitment to their jobs, that *individuals* in one group report as much commitment to their jobs as *individuals* in another, and that the relationship between how *individuals* rank their leaders and how they rank their own commitment is consistent across the three groups.

The data do *not* show that *groups* with more highly ranked leaders have more committed members. In fact, if one were to draw any conclusions about groups from these data, it would have to be that there is an *inverse* relationship between leadership and commitment. This will be discussed further in the next section.

Conclusions drawn from data describing the individual as the unit of analysis refer to individual characteristics. Therefore, as demonstrated, drawing conclusions about group characteristics from individual data can be grossly misleading. The extent to which data collected from individuals inaccurately reflect relationships among groups depends on the actual distribution of individual responses within and between groups for the variables involved. As will be shown, in some cases, similar conclusions will be reached with either individual or group-level data. In those cases, the covariation among the variables that characterize groups is similar to the covariation among variables when they are used to characterize individuals. For example, one could discover that groups with highly rated leaders have high levels of commitment and also that individuals who rate their group leaders highly report high levels of individual commitment. This is not necessarily so, however, and researchers must guard against drawing conclusions about one unit of analysis with data that are based on the other.

AGGREGATING INDIVIDUAL RESPONSES
WITHIN GROUPS

It is common practice in family, group and organizational research to obtain data for these collectives by aggregating the responses of the individuals within each family, group or organization. In this way, the collectives serve as the units of analysis. Although this practice does establish the collective as the unit of analysis, and thus solves the problem described in the prior section, additional theoretical and empirical problems are created.

To return to our example from small group research, the practice of aggregating the responses of group members to characterize a group implies an important assumption. It assumes that the variation of individual responses within the groups is smaller than that between the groups. In other words, the practice implies that the individual responses are more a function of group membership than of individual characteristics.

Figure 1 can be used to illustrate the problems created when this assumption does not hold. If the individual responses were aggregated by obtaining averages on the leadership and commitment measures for each group, the group data would be plotted as indicated by the three x's. It is evident that this strategy would produce a negative relationship between X and Y, using the group as the unit of analysis, although using the individual as the unit of analysis would have produced a positive relationship. It appears, from these data, that the relationship between leadership and commitment is positive for individuals, but negative for groups.

The discrepancy is caused, in part, by the fact that there is greater within-group variation than between-group variation. In other words, the characteristics of the individual have more influence on the individual responses than do the characteristics of the group.

To illustrate the effects of the source of variation, Figure 2 shows the same general pattern of responses, but in this case the within-group variation is smaller than the between-group variation. Here, an analysis of the relationship using the individual as the unit of analysis would provide the same results

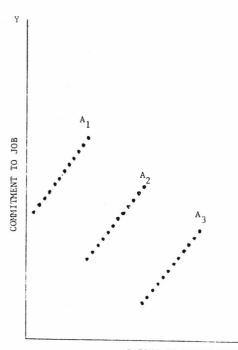

Y

COMMITMENT TO JOB

A_1

A_2

A_3

RATING OF LEADERSHIP   X

Stylized Distribution of Values for Individuals (N=36)

in Three Work Groups (A_1, A_2, A_3)

FIGURE 2

as that using the group as the unit of analysis. This illustrates a situation in which the group characteristics have a greater impact on responses than do individual characteristics. Note that within each group, as in Figure 1, the relationship between X and Y remains positive, although overall the relationship is negative for both the group and the individual units of analysis. At the individual level, this diagram represents a classical suppression effect (not to be confused with interaction). Although X and Y are negatively related, if the effects of A (group membership) were partialed, or held constant, the relationship between X and Y would be positive. In Figure 1, in contrast, A has little effect, and the relationship between X and Y is positive whether A is partialed or not.

Figure 3 is an example of a situation in which, again, an analysis based on the group and individual units of analysis

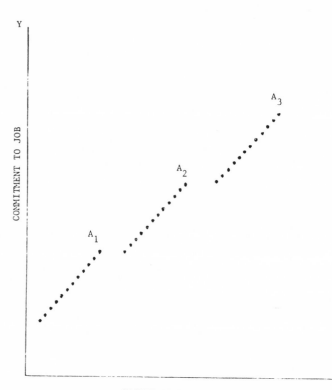

RATING OF LEADERSHIP   X

Stylized Distribution of Values for Individuals (N=36)

in Three Work Groups (A_1, A_2, A_3)

FIGURE 3

would provide essentially the same results. As in Figure 2, the within-group variation is smaller than the between-group variation. But, unlike Figure 2, there is no suppression effect. The relationship between X and Y at the individual level of analysis is the same with or without A partialed, or held constant.

The above illustrations show that aggregating individual data to determine relationships at the group level can lead to error unless conclusions are appropriately tempered. In some cases, as shown in Figure 1, aggregation is difficult to justify. The following section furthers the discussion by providing examples of discrepancies between individual and group covariation in an actual data set.

AN EXAMPLE

The following data were collected from 331 members of 53 workgroups in 22 different human service organizations. The data were collected to determine the relationship between the commitment of human service workers to the jobs they perform as members of small workgroups and a number of variables that describe the workgroups, the workers, the tasks performed by the workers, and the organization within which the workgroup exists. A major objective of the study was to examine the relationship between the commitment of workgroup members and the ratings given workgroup leaders.

The data were first analyzed using the individual as the unit of analysis. Individual responses were then aggregated by workgroup and the same analyses repeated using the group as the unit of analyses.

Table 2 shows the zero-order correlation coefficients between commitment and variables describing the workgroup, the worker, the tasks performed by the workers, the organization within which the workgroup exists, and the workgroup leadership.

The first column reports the correlations when using the individual as the unit of analysis and the second, using the group as the unit of analysis. Some variable values would be unchanged by averaging individual data within groups. These

Table 2

Zero-order Correlation Coefficients for the Relationships
Between Commitment and Predictors

Unit of Analysis

Variable	Individual (N=331)	Group (N=53)
Workgroup size	.04	.05
Organization budget	.03	.09
Organization age	.42**	.54**
Workgroup age	-.02	-.14
Years in organization	-.01	-.07
Years experience	-.04	-.13
Age of worker	.34**	.49**
Sex of worker	-.10	-.27*
Education of worker	-.20**	-.24
Salary of worker	-.12**	-.23
Leadership rating	.50**	.62**
Conflict rating	-.43**	-.46**
Ambiguity rating	-.59**	-.67**
Skill variety	.08	.21
Task identity	.30**	.41**
Task significance	.31**	.45**
Residential services	.10	.35**
Residential and outpatient	-.04	-.25

*p<.05
**p<.01

would include workgroup size, organization budget, organization age, workgroup age, residential services, and residential and outpatient. The variables, residential services, and residential and outpatient, are dummy coded, and together represent a three level nominal variable, type of service. The three types of human services delivered by these workgroups are outpatient services, residential services, and residential and outpatient services. Outpatient services was chosen as the reference level. These dummy variables and the workgroup and organization variables listed above would be unchanged by averaging within workgroups since all members of a given workgroup would have equal values for these variables.

The remaining variables describe individual workgroup members and would change when averaged. The leadership, conflict, and ambiguity ratings were based on scales completed individually that, respectively, evaluated the leader of the workgroup, and the conflict and the ambiguity experienced by workgroup members in performing the jobs. The skill and task variables refer to the nature of the skills and tasks required to perform the job.

Note that the design used to obtain these data is a combination of the most common design in social work small group research, the survey, and the quasi-experimental design shown in Table 1. Using the individual unit of analysis, strategies A-2 and A-3, the relationships among variables characterizing individuals are examined. In addition, groups of nonrandomly assigned individuals under three conditions (residential services, residential and outpatient, and outpatient services) are compared. Using the group unit of analysis, strategies B-2 and B-3, the relationships among characteristics of a sample of groups are examined, and groups of nonrandomly assigned groups under several conditions (residential services, residential and outpatient, and outpatient services) are compared.

An evaluation of the two columns of correlation coefficients reveals higher correlation coefficients for the group data regardless of whether the predictor describes the organization, the workgroup or the worker. Also, the directions of the relationships are unchanged. These data are similar to the stylized pattern of responses shown in Figure 3. The higher correlations are a function of the decrease in error variation that results from averaging data in patterns similar to Figure 3.

For eight of the variables, correlations are more than doubled when the group is used as the unit of analysis. Because of the decrease in the degrees of freedom, however, in only two of those cases, sex and residential services, would conclusions based upon inferential tests of significance differ between the individual and the group data. It is interesting to note that one variable, sex, would be changed in value by aggregating (coded 0 for females and 1 for males, a group average then represents the proportion of males in the group), but the other, residential services (coded 0 or 1, all members of a single workgroup would have the same value), would not be changed.

Multiple regression analyses of the individual and group data, moreover, show a similar number of discrepancies and, in addition, the direction of the differences are not consistent across all variables. As shown in Table 3, there are six vari-

Table 3

Regression Equations for Predicting Commitment

Variable	Unit of Analysis	
	Individual (N=331)	Group (N=53)
Intercept	59.95	73.26
Workgroup size	-.35**	-.74
Organization budget	.00	.00
Organization age	.12**	.08*
Workgroup age	.10	.10
Years in organization	.25	.22
Years experience	-.40	-.84
Age of worker	.05	-.05
Sex of worker	-2.64	-2.61
Education of worker	-2.41*	-7.83**
Salary of worker	.19	.40
Leadership rating	.35**	.36*
Conflict rating	-.15	-.14
Ambiguity rating	-.58**	-.96**
Skill variety	.36	1.45*
Task identity	.13	.03
Task significance	.22	.91
Residential services	3.79	-5.51
Residential and outpatient	5.29**	5.61*
R^2	.57**	.87**

*$p<.05$
**$p<.01$

ables for which the group-level regression coefficients are at least twice as large as the individual-level regression coefficients. Task identity, in contrast, provides an example of an individual-level regression coefficient that is four times as large as the group-level regression coefficient. Some of these seven variables had values that were altered by averaging within groups and some were not.

One of the coefficients, for residential services, changed signs. This indicates that the adjusted mean commitment level for individuals delivering residential services was higher than that of individuals delivering outpatient services, but the adjusted mean commitment level of groups delivering residential services was *lower* than that of groups delivering outpatient services!

Decisions regarding the significance of relationships between commitment and the specific predictors would have varied in two instances. Workgroup size was significantly related to commitment at the individual level but not at the group level, and skill variety was significantly related to commitment at the group level but not at the individual level. Not only, then, are there discrepancies in the descriptive statistics as described above, but there exists the additional problem of discrepancies in conclusions based upon inferential tests of significance for both the correlation coefficients and the regression coefficients.

CONCLUSIONS

The paper has raised a general question concerning the differences between using the individual as the unit of analysis (Strategy A) and using the group as the unit of analysis (Strategy B) in small group research. It has been argued that observed relationships among the characteristics of individuals cannot always be generalized successfully to the characteristics of groups of those individuals. A separate but related problem concerns the appropriateness of aggregating the responses of individuals within a group for analyses using the group as the unit of analysis.

The most common strategy used in studying small group phenomena, as indicated by the published research in five major social work journals, is a survey of individuals in one or more group conditions (Strategy A-2). An example of a survey of 331 individuals in 53 different workgroups showed major discrepancies between results analyzed with the individual and with the group units of analysis. Discrepancies appeared in both correlation and regression analyses and were distributed over variables characterizing both the workgroup (workgroup size, residential services) and the individual (years of experience, education of worker, salary of worker, sex, skill variety, task identity and task significance). These results suggest that the practices of analyzing individual variation for the purposes of drawing conclusions about groups and of characterizing a group by aggregating characteristics of the members of the group are questionable. Although not designed to address the issue of the appropriate unit of analysis, recent research by Toseland, Rivas, and

Chapman, (1984) has also shown discrepancies between results using groups values and those using individual values aggregated by group.

It is suggested that additional theoretical and empirical attention be given to the issue of the appropriate unit of analysis in small group research. In the interim, it would be prudent for researchers who gather data using the individual as the unit of analysis to refrain from generalizing results to group characteristics. The general tendency among researchers to fail to clearly and specifically distinguish between the analyses of covariation of individual characteristics in group situations and the analyses of covariation of group characteristics signals the presence of confusion over that difference, both theoretically and empirically.

REFERENCES

Davis, Larry E., "Racial Composition of Groups," *Social Work* 24(3), 1979, pp. 208–213.

Feldman, Ronald A., and Timothy E. Caplinger, "Social Work Experience and Client Behavioral Change: A Multivariate Analysis of Process and Outcome," *Journal of Social Service Research* 1(1), 1977, pp. 5–33.

Glisson, Charles, "Trends in Social Work Research: Substantive and Methodological Implications for Doctoral Curricula," presented to the annual meeting of the Group for the Advancement of Doctoral Education (GADE), University of Alabama, October 10, 1983.

Glisson, Charles and Patricia Y. Martin, "Productivity and Efficiency in Human Service Organizations as Related to Structure, Size, and Age," *Academy of Management Journal* 23(1), 1980, pp. 21–37.

Lawrence, Harry and Claude L. Walter, "Testing a Behavioral Approach with Groups," *Social Work* 23(2), 1978, pp. 127–133.

Rose, Sheldon D., "How Group Attributes Relate to Outcome in Behavior Group Therapy," *Social Work Research and Abstracts* 17(3), 1981, pp. 25–29.

Schopler, Janice H., and Maeda J. Galinsky, "When Groups Go Wrong," *Social Work* 26 (5), 1981, pp. 424–429.

Segal, Uma A., "Micro-Behaviors in Group Decision-Making: An Exploratory Study," *Journal of Social Service Research* 5(1/2), 1982, pp. 1–14.

Toseland, Ronald W., Robert F. Rivas, and Dennis Chapman, "An Evaluation of Decision-Making Methods in Task Groups," *Social Work* 29(4), 1984, pp. 339–346.

Developmental Research
for Task-Centered Group Work
with Chronic Mental Patients

Charles Garvin

ABSTRACT. A project to develop and evaluate a task-centered group work technology for use with chronic mental patients is described. Details are presented on the evolution of the project and the rationale for it. These include staff selection and training, member recruitment and preparation, group composition, the specification of group procedures, and the creation of evaluation instruments. Future stages of project development are identified.

This paper reports the progress of a project currently being conducted at the School of Social Work of the University of Michigan. The project aims to develop and evaluate a task-centered group work technology for use with chronic mental patients. This project is an example of developmental research which Thomas (1984: 23) defines as " . . . consisting of those methods by which the social technology of human service is analyzed, designed, created, and evaluated." Thomas indicates that the phases of such research are "analysis, development (which also includes design), and evaluation, each of which has its activities and steps." It should be noted that this project was not conceived as completely following Thomas's model but rather as a parallel effort drawing from his principles but not necessarily in full compliance with them.

The project is currently in a pilot phase. This paper describes what has been accomplished thus far as well as the plans for subsequent phases. This pilot phase involved devel-

Charles Garvin, PhD, is Professor of Social Work, School of Social Work, University of Michigan, Ann Arbor, Michigan.

oping and implementing a task-centered group work technology and a series of instruments to evaluate it. The subsequent phase will involve the utilization of this technology with a large enough sample to evaluate its effectiveness. That phase, therefore, will necessarily involve a control group design, a refinement of instrumentation, and a comprehensive analysis of a wide range of data. The background of the project, the way that group members have been recruited, the training of the group workers, the preparation of members, the specification of group work procedures, the creation and selection of evaluation instruments, and the way that planning will occur for the next phase will now be described.

In task-centered practice, the client is helped to define his or her problems, generate goals that will ameliorate the problem, and choose and carry out *tasks* in order to attain these goals. In task-centered group work, the group members agree to help each other to define problems, choose goals and tasks, and carry out tasks. Task-centered practice is intended to be short term; both the individual and group models anticipate about twelve sessions. Further information regarding task-centered group work can be found in discussions by Garvin (1974, 1984).

PROJECT BACKGROUND

The steps leading to this project began over ten years ago when the author became acquainted with task-centered casework (Reid and Epstein, 1972). He indicated to Reid and Epstein, its creators, that the purposes of their technology could be accomplished through the application of group processes and then proceeded to generate a model for this approach (Garvin, 1974). Shortly after the appearance of this article, Reid and Epstein carried out empirical tests of task-centered group work with twelve groups. They found support for its effectiveness with children's groups in schools but not with a group of women with "reactive depression" (Garvin, Reid, and Epstein, 1976).

During the ten years following the Reid-Epstein research a number of other empirically based projects were conducted that examined the effectiveness of task-centered group work with such populations as the elderly, delinquents, and mental patients. Based on these works, the model was updated in 1984 (Garvin, 1984). This update indicates that task-centered group work is still at an early stage of development as a truly empirically based approach. The work done by others *suggests* its effectiveness but does not yet adequately demonstrate it. The technology employed in each project was not well specified and the research designs that were utilized are deficient in some respect in each case. Such deficiencies are typical of early stages of developmental research and are, themselves, limited by such stages. Nevertheless, sufficient work has now been done to serve as the basis for a rigorous test of the model with a selected population.

A number of target client populations were considered in terms of several criteria: the appropriateness of the model for the population; the accessibility of the population (likelihood of agency cooperation, likelihood of sufficient referrals for groups); the degree to which more effective services for the population would be responsive to a pressing social need; and the availability of graduate social work students in the agency to help with the groups.

On the basis of these criteria, work with the chronic mentally ill living in the community seemed appropriate. This population is often responsive to structured group experiences (Goldstein, Sprafkin, and Gershaw, 1976). Because of the policy of deinstitutionalization, every community mental health program is flooded with clients who tax its services. The local community mental health center was no exception and reacted quickly and positively. A large number of social work students are placed for training in this agency. And, finally, at least one effort to use task-centered groups with this population met with positive results (Newcome, 1984).

The goal of developing a project to contribute to the rehabilitation of chronic mental patients is fairly modest. It is not to provide a "cure" but rather to add another intervention to the series of effective programs that each client uses. Intervention will be deemed successful if it helps clients to engage in constructive activities with others, learn to make plans for themselves that are more realistic than is presently the case, and come to see themselves as capable of taking actions on their own behalf to a greater degree.

The Community Mental Health Center in a middle sized midwestern city, in responding favorably to a proposal to jointly sponsor this pilot project, agreed to the following: they would assign staff and students to work with the project and would allocate a portion of their time to it; they would assign an agency administrator as liaison to the project; they would supply program funds for the groups; and they would cooperate in referring clients to groups.

Work began with a group of paid staff and students in October, 1984. After some inevitable shifts, the staff consisted of five employees and three students. In addition, two faculty from the School joined the project as well as a doctoral student who was fulfilling his requirement for a research internship.

INITIAL PLANNING AND TRAINING

The first activity was to train the staff in task-centered concepts. To accomplish this, staff was assigned to read the most recent article about this approach (Garvin, 1984). Subsequent discussions were based on the article. We planned to further orient the staff to the model by involving them in detailed session by session planning for each group. Despite the fact that all staff had MSW degrees, it was later learned that several had not received much basic group work training. As a result, several sessions devoted to basic group work principles were conducted. It is possible that if all staff have group work training, the quality of service may be higher. But we were restricted to what could be obtained from the agency's existing resources for this project and hoped that close supervision and ongoing training could reasonably substitute for fully trained group workers.

After the orientation period, the staff engaged in an analysis of the specific types of clients who might be recruited for our groups. They listed all the types of chronic mental patients served by the agency and discussed each in terms of the appropriateness of task-centered work, the size of the client pool, and the agency's priorities. Based upon these criteria, four groups were formed, each serving a different sub-population and each having a purpose drawn from the agency's service goals for the type of client in question. The four groups were the following:

1. A group composed of clients who are among the agency's lowest functioning yet who are capable of agreeing to attend a group and for whom there is a reasonable likelihood of attendance with encouragement and reinforcement. These clients, however, have difficulty acting appropriately in social situations and have minimal social skills. This was viewed as a "pre-task-centered group" as the purposes for the group include helping the members understand such concepts as "goals." It was also planned that the member tasks would all be carried out within the group.
2. A group composed primarily of clients diagnosed as schizophrenic who are unemployed and who spend most of their daytime hours alone and usually at home. These hours are often spent watching television or sleeping. Some of these clients may also be enrolled in a sheltered workshop program but the rest of their time is likely to be spent in solitary, undemanding pursuits. The purpose of the group is to improve their use of leisure time in the direction of activities that are more social, cultivate new interests, enhance their self-esteem, or contribute to vocational planning.
3. A group composed of clients who are similar to those described in (2) but who also have substance abuse problems. The staff suspect that some of their use of substances is related to self-medication to ameliorate the side effects of drugs prescribed for their mental illnesses.
4. A group composed of women who, in addition to the social limitations found in the clients identified as part of the second group, are "trapped" in family situations that are highly stressful.

RECRUITMENT AND SCREENING

After deciding on the above purposes for the groups, a process to recruit members was established. The staff determined that case managers in the agency would wish to refer clients but would not do so because of their large caseloads if the referral process were time consuming. Therefore, they were only required to complete a form that asked the client's name, case number, address, phone, and for which group the referral was intended. These forms were distributed at an agency-wide staff meeting at which general information was given on the program as well as specific details regarding the four groups.

When the referral was received, a worker assigned to the intended group interviewed the case manager on the phone for more information. This information was to be used for purposes of group composition as well as helping members to choose goals and tasks. More referrals were received than "slots" in the groups. When a referral was rejected, it was indicated that more clients might be accommodated in future stages of the project if there was success in an application for funding.

The telephone interview questions included client's psychiatric diagnosis, use of substances, living situation, previous group experience, treatment currently received, employment status, type of peer interaction, presence of bizarre behavior, problems in social functioning, use of leisure time, and mental status. This latter item was used to secure information on how logical were the client's thought processes, how reality oriented were the client's cognitions, whether the client was overly concrete or abstract in his or her thinking, and whether other dysfunctional thought patterns were present. The workers were also asked how they anticipated the clients benefitting from the group.

When this information was secured, it was used for the process of group composition. The lowest functioning group was to be allocated about six members and the others about eight. About two more members were allocated to each group so as to allow for attrition. In general a balance of men and women (except in the all-women's group) and of blacks and whites was sought. The group composition procedure described by Garvin (1981) was employed. This involved charting salient member characteristics to avoid any one member being extremely different from all other members in reference to significant attributes.

Following the composition procedure, the project staff interviewed each potential client in order to ascertain the client's willingness to participate. They also followed the plan prescribed for task-centered groups in which clients begin the process of goal identification prior to the first meeting in order to accelerate the work in view of its short term nature. Another reason for this is evidence that members who are prepared for groups are more likely to invest themselves in the group and to achieve their goals (Garvin, 1981: 78–80). Clients were told about task-centered work and the purposes of the group and asked if they wished to be in a group with that approach and intent. During the pre-group interview, client questions about the group were answered and their feelings about joining were discussed. All interviewed clients agreed to participate at that point.

SPECIFYING GROUP PROCEDURES

One of the major objectives of developmental research is the design of the intervention (Thomas, 1984: 151–190). As stated earlier, one of the defects of evaluations of task-centered group work is that the intervention has not been adequately specified. A good deal of procedural detail about the conduct of task-centered groups has been provided in a recent article (Garvin, 1984). That article was intended to serve as a basis for task-centered work with a wide variety of populations and, therefore, necessitated a high level of abstraction. In this project, the abstractions had to be reduced to very concrete levels.

For this reason, we sought in the current project to plan the procedures in as much detail as possible and then to monitor their implementation. The monitoring will allow the investigators to describe not only what was planned but whether or not each aspect of the plan was implemented and whether changes were made in the plan during implementation. It was decided, however, not to plan the entire series of sessions but only the first two or three. The reason for this was that is was uncertain how members would respond to the initial stage of the group; it was necessary to take this into consideration in the detailed planning of later sessions.

An example of the type of procedural guidelines being developed is the following plan for the second meeting of group #2:

1. Development of individual goals.

The idea of the "time line" that was presented at the previous meeting is reviewed. Each member reviews his or her previous day and with the help of the group creates a time line on a sheet of paper that has been made available. Members are asked whether that day was a "typical" one. If not, a more typical day may be substituted. The member is then asked what might be one way in which his or her use of leisure time on that day might have been enhanced (i.e., what is something he or she would have wished to do that would have been the way he or she wished to spend time). Members give feedback to each other (with help of the workers) in the form of suggestions. Members are asked whether this use of time is the one that they wish to make their goal for the group experience. If not, with the help of time lines other types of goals are considered. The object, however, is to create a goal in the form of a time line.

How the member wishes to spend his or her time may not necessarily be within his or her competency at the time. The purpose is to identify some way that the member will wish to use time at the end of the process. There may be several intermediate steps in the form of tasks; these can be placed on a time line also.

It is estimated that the above process may take 10–15 minutes per member so that the group will have to be subdivided into two subgroups of about four members. With this approach, the process will take about an hour. The workers should try to create two subgroups with about equal distribution of members who will approach this process slowly to make it likely that the two groups will finish in about the same time.

2. "Leisure time experience."

Since members will have been "working," the last 15–30 minutes should be spent in some way that is reinforcing. This should be in the form of refreshments and a game. The game that we recommend is "Leisure Time Trivia" (developed for this project). The group is divided into two subgroups. The questions are illustrated by the following: name three objects that are necessary for a baseball game; name one movie now playing in Ann Arbor.

3. Evaluation.

The meeting should conclude with some discussion of feelings about the group and how things are going. The plan for the next meeting is described in which members affirm whether or not they wish to commit themselves to the goals chosen this week and then begin to create tasks.

A form has been devised that workers complete after each meeting. They record whether or not they followed procedures and how they may have been modified. The form lists each meeting portion by its number on the meeting plan and asks for a rating of the portion and a description of any modification. The rating indicates whether the portion occurred as planned and accomplished its purposes; whether minor problems arose that did not interfere with this; whether modifications were made to achieve the purposes; whether the portion met with major problems; or whether that portion of the plan was aborted.

In addition, the meeting report form requests the names of members present and absent, details about critical incidents, and questions and problems for team discussion.

EVALUATION INSTRUMENTS

One major problem with which the investigators struggled was a lack of resources to develop and pretest many types of instruments. The greatest resource lack relates to the group leadership itself. The groups were each co-led by two workers. These eight workers consisted of five regular staff and three social work students. Each regular staff member had many additional assignments even though some reduction of their workload occurred to make project participation possible. Each social work student had other assignments. Every instrument required additional staff time. The limits of staff tolerance for work overload was reached when a minimal rather than optimal set of instruments was presented to them.

Nevertheless, the measures employed were chosen with careful consideration given to the rationale behind task-centered work. This rationale is that clients enter service to resolve problems in social functioning. To accomplish this, they choose to attain specified goals. To attain goals, they try to accomplish tasks. Instruments utilized in the pilot phase related to the measurement of problems in functioning, goal attainment, and task accomplishment.

To examine the extent of problems in social functioning relevant to project objectives, a personal inventory was completed by each group member at the first and last group meetings. This inventory utilized items from scales devised by Schneider and Struening (1983) and by Katz and Lyerly (1963). The former scale was tested by its authors for interrater reliability, factorial validity, invariance, and interval consistency reliability on a sample of 173 community agency and 982 state hospital clients. The latter was examined for validity by its creators through concurrent ratings by patients and relatives as well as for internal consistency and stability of measure across populations.

The inventory we used consisted of 31 items, each rated on a five point scale. One subset of items relates to self-care such as responsibility for clothing, medical appointments, medication, money management, meal preparation, and housework. Another subset relates to social activities such as visiting friends, entertaining at home, taking courses, volunteering in community agencies, and handling tensions between self and others. A third subset relates to such leisure time activities as reading, listening to music, going to movies, engaging in crafts, sports, library use, and walking.

Reid (1978) has developed a rating system for problem assessment that is appropriate for this project. Reid's system provides for a rating of problem reduction in which the rater can choose from a series of scales the one that "fits" the type of problem selected. Some scales relate to problems specified in quantitative formats while others can be used when the problem specification needs to be more qualitative. The investigators were unable to pretest a form of that instrument because of the lack of staff resources. They plan on testing the feasibility and validity of this instrument in a subsequent project.

Goal attainment is being measured through the use of goal attainment scales (Kiresuk and Garwick, 1979: 412–421). While some criticisms have been levelled against this measure on statistical grounds, there does not appear to be any other instrument that is as valid for measuring individually chosen goals.

A problem that was encountered in the utilization of the goal attainment scale was the process of specifying levels of goal achievement greater and lesser than the expected one. The group workers on this project believe that this population of clients would find it a negative and confusing experience to select such levels of goal attainment. For this reason, the workers themselves identified the levels once a contract on goals had been negotiated with the member.

To measure task accomplishment, a series of items was incorporated into the weekly progress notes that staff are routinely required by agency policy to complete. These items consist of a statement of the task undertaken that week; the ordinal position of the task (first, second, third, and so on) if the client has undertaken several tasks (or subtasks); the obstacles the client has identified to task accomplishment; the plan for overcoming such obstacles; who suggested the task; and, finally, ratings of the client's commitment to the task and the degree of task accomplishment.

As indicated, if resources were available the investigators would have devised and utilized a number of other measures. These would include interviews with significant others regarding observations of client progress as well as behavioral ratings of client in-group behaviors. In addition, it would have been of value to understand better how group-level variables are affected by task-centered interventions. This would have required measures of group cohesiveness (beyond attendance records), group structures such as communication patterns and changing roles, and group problem solving. Another topic of interest is the group's development patterns. It is hoped that the subsequent phase of this project will bring sufficient funding for these types of research activities to be conducted.

NEXT STEPS

At the completion of this pilot project, the procedures that were employed will be analyzed; this will lead to a revised model for work with the chronic mentally ill. The outcome data will also be analyzed to see if it provides sufficient information to serve as a basis for outcome measurement of task-centered group work. Where gaps exist, the investigators will seek to identify other measures that might be employed in the subsequent project. Based upon this and a review of the literature on group interventions with similar populations, we hope to develop a sound design for a full field test of the model—one that will be attractive to potential funding resources. We believe from our experiences thus far that we are creating an intervention program that can make a significant contribution to the amelioration of a pressing social problem.

REFERENCES

Garvin, C. Task-centered group work. *Social Service Review.* 1974, 48, 494–507.

Garvin, C., Reid, W., & Epstein, L. Task-centered group work. In R.W. Roberts and H. Northen (Eds.) *Theoretical approaches to social work with small groups.* New York: Columbia University Press, 1976.

Garvin, C. *Contemporary group work.* Englewood Cliffs, N.J.: Prentice-Hall, 1981.

Garvin, C. Task-centered group work. In A. Fortune (Ed.) *Task-centered practice with families and groups.* New York: Springer, 1984.

Goldstein, A., Sprafkin, R.P., & Gershaw, N.J. *Skill training for community living: applying structured learning therapy.* New York: Pergamon, 1976.

Katz, M.A. and Lyerly, S.B. Methods for measuring adjustment and social behavior in the community: rationale, description, discriminative validity, and scale development. *Psychological Reports.* 1963, 13, 503–535.

Kiresuk, T. & Garwick, G. Basic goal attainment procedures. In B. Compton & B. Galaway (Eds.) *Social work processes. 2nd Ed.* Homewood, Ill.: Dorsey Press, 1979.

Newcome, K. Task-centered group work with the chronically mentally ill in day treatment. In A. Fortune (Ed.) *Task-centered practice with families and groups.* New York: Springer, 1984.

Reid, W. & Epstein, L. *Task-centered casework.* New York: Columbia University Press, 1972.

Reid. W. *The task-centered system.* New York: Columbia University Press, 1978.

Schneider. L.C. and Struening, E.L. SLOF: a behavioral rating scale for assessing the mentally ill. *Social Work Research and Abstracts.* 1983, 19, 9–21.

Thomas, E.J. *Designing Interventions for the helping professions.* Beverly Hills: Sage, 1984.

Meta-Analysis:
Statistical Considerations and Applications in Small Group Treatment Research

Steven H. Tallant

INTRODUCTION

Traditional qualitative literature reviews have long played a central role in scientific development. However, within the past decade there has been an increased awareness and application of quantitative methods for reviewing research in which data from different studies are statistically combined. Generally referred to as meta-analysis, a typical meta-analytic package consists of techniques for combining probabilities across studies, estimating the average size of treatment effect, determining the stability of results, and identifying factors that moderate the outcome of separate studies (Strube & Hartman, 1983). The use of meta-analytic procedures as either an adjunctive method to or as a replacement for the qualitative review method has been both highly acclaimed and criticized (Cook & Leviton, 1980; Cooper, 1979; Cooper & Arkin, 1981; Eysenck, 1978; Glass, McGraw, & Smith, 1981).

On one hand, advocates of meta-analytic methods have criticized the qualitative methods of review on three principal grounds: (1) that relevant information is ignored in favor of a simplistic box count of the number of studies in which a par-

Captain Steven H. Tallant, PhD, is Director, Alcoholism Rehabilitation Center, USAF Medical Center, Scott AFB, Illinois.

The author expresses appreciation and gratitude to Professor Ronald Serlin, Department of Educational Sciences, University of Wisconsin-Madison, for statistical consultation in preparing this paper.

ticular relationship is and is not statistically significant; (2) that the sample of studies for review often contains important biases; and (3) that box counts ignore statistical interactions (Glass, 1978; Glass & Smith, 1979; Smith and Glass, 1977). These advocates believe meta-analytic methods allow for a more systematic and objective analysis of all research studies which bear data on a given issue.

On the other hand, the methodological problems involved in combining quantitative results are formidable and well documented in the literature (Rosenthal, 1978; Eysenck, 1978; Mintz, 1983; Wilson & Rachman, 1983; Nurius, 1984). Glass and his colleagues (Glass, McGraw, & Smith, 1981) have noted three primary areas in which meta-analytic methods have been criticized. The first criticism refers to the conceptual and methodological appropriateness of comparing or combining studies with different measures, samples, designs, or constructs. The second criticism refers to the use of studies with poor designs. Finally, the pooling of studies has been criticized for violating assumptions of independence of data (for a complete discussion regarding these criticisms refer to Glass, McGraw, & Smith, 1981 and Nurius, 1984).

Unfortunately, while there has been a recent proliferation of articles pertaining to the potential uses and abuses of meta-analytic methods, there appear to be two issues which have been generally ignored in the literature. First, while critics have pointed out the methodological problems associated with meta-analysis there has been little discussion regarding the statistical problems associated with combining quantitative data from different studies. Second, the literature has focused primarily upon the use of meta-analytic procedures as a means of conducting quantitative literature reviews. The value of utilizing meta-analytic methods as a planned, adjunctive statistical method in the course of developmental research has not been generally recognized.

The purpose of this paper is threefold. First, a review of the meta-analytic procedure most often utilized in the behavioral sciences will be presented. Second, the statistical problems associated with this procedure are examined. Third, the potential value of applying meta-analytic methods in small group treatment research is discussed.

THE GLASS EFFECT SIZE ESTIMATOR

The term meta-analysis, coined by Glass in 1976, is used ambiguously throughout the literature. On one hand, it is used as a generic term referring to the use of several formal analytic procedures for combining results across several studies (Cook & Gruder, 1978; Cooper, 1979; Cook and Leviton, 1980; Pillermer and Light, 1980; Leviton and Cook, 1981). On the other hand, it is often used to refer to one specific data synthesizing technique, namely, the technique developed by Glass to estimate effect size (Glass, 1976; Smith & Glass, 1977; Glass, McGraw, & Smith, 1981; Kraemer, 1983, Nurius, 1984).

For the purpose of this paper, the term meta-analysis will refer to the specific technique developed by Glass. The rationale is as follows:

1. A discussion and critique of the full range of all data synthesizing techniques and methods is beyond the scope of this paper:
2. Glass's estimator of effect size has been applied extensively in the behavioral sciences and is the most applicable for small group treatment research;
3. The bulk of the methodological and statistical criticisms of meta-analysis has been with the Glass estimator.

The effects size (ES) of Glass is a numerical index of the magnitude of the treatment typically calculated by subtracting the mean of the study control group (MC) from the mean of the treatment group (MT) and dividing that difference by the standard deviation of the control group (SDC). Therefore:

$$ES = (MT - MC) / SDC$$

As a standard score, the ES index reflects by how many standard deviation units one group mean is different from another. A positive ES indicates the treatment group scored higher on the measure in question; a negative ES indicates the control group scored higher. The common range of effect sizes in social and behavioral research is from -1 to $+1$ (Cohen, 1977) encompassing 68% of the sample (34% on each side of the control group mean). Therefore, an $ES = +1$

would indicate a person at the mean of the control group would be expected to rise to the 84th percentile of the control group (or fall to the 16th percentile if ES = −1) after the experimental manipulation (Smith and Glass, 1977). The unit of analysis then becomes the effect size rather than the original measure. An average effect size is computed to obtain a single precise quantitative statistic representing all studies under review. Assuming normal distribution a Z-table is used to translate the score of the average person in the treatment group.

Many different techniques can be applied to Glass's effect size estimator. The literature is replete with examples. They include generating a single precise summary statistic with a confidence interval, blocking techniques, correlational synthesis, regression analysis, and cumulative time studies (Glass, 1976; Smith and Glass, 1977; Glass and Smith, 1977; Glass et al., 1981; Berk, 1981, De Silva, 1981).

Statistical Problems Associated with the Glass Estimator

Effect Size Estimator

As noted previously, Glass's estimator of effect size is ES = XT − XC / SDC. Glass proposed that the use of the standard deviation of the control group be used to standardize the mean difference. His argument was that pooling two variances could lead to different standardized values at the identical mean difference within an experiment where several treatments were compared to a control condition.

The use of the standard deviation of the control group has been criticized by several statisticians (Kraemer, 1983; Hedges, 1981; Hedges, 1982, Hunter, Schmidt, & Jackson, 1982). These statisticians all agree that the pooled-within group variance is a better sample estimator.

Because the statistical analysis using the effect size typically involves the use of a t or F test for difference between the groups, Hedges (1981) examined the difference between the pooled-within group variance and the control group variance based upon the assumptions of the t and F test. Hedges was able to derive the properties of both estimators of d (effect size) based on the *assumptions*:

$$Y_{ij}^E \sim N(\mu_i^E, \sigma_i^2),$$

$$j = 1, \ldots, n_i^E, \, i = 1, \ldots, k,$$

and

$$Y_{ij}^C \sim N(\mu_i^C, \sigma_i^2),$$

$$j = 1, \ldots, n_i^C, \, i = 1, \ldots, k.$$

effect size:

$$\pounds_i = \frac{\mu_i^E - \mu_i^C}{\sigma_i}$$

By utilizing these assumptions, Hedges found the distributions of each estimator directly from the non-central t-distribution. In particular

$$g_i \sqrt{n_i^E n_i^C / (n_i^E + n_i^C)}$$

is distributed as a non-central t-variable with non-centrality parameter

$$\pounds \sqrt{n_i^E n_i^C / (n_i^E + n_i^C)}$$

and degree of freedom equal to N_i^C- or $n_i^E + n_i^C - 2$. Hedges concludes that the distributions of each estimator are identical except for the number of degrees of freedom used to estimate the standard deviation. This bias approaches zero when the number of degrees of freedom used to estimate the standard deviation is large, but it can be substantial when the number of degrees of freedom is small. As a result, Hedges states that the pooled-within group variance should be used.

In addition to these statistical considerations, Hunter and his colleagues (Hunter et al., 1981) note that most published reports have a value for t or F and therefore permit the computation of the d statistic using the within-group variance. However, few reports present standard deviations in which case the effect size using control-group only standard deviations can not be computed.

Bias of the d Statistic (Effect Size)

After the d statistic has been calculated for a given study, most meta-analysts have not clearly distinguished sample estimates of effect size from the population parameter that they wished to estimate (Hedges, 1982). For example, Glass cites 26 articles which performed meta-analysis; none differentiated the sample estimate from the population parameter (Glass et al., 1981).

Hedges (1981, 1982), Kraemer (1983), and Hunter (1982) all emphasize that the effect size is a sample statistic and therefore has a sampling distribution of its own. They concur with Hedges regarding the unbiased estimator of £. This unbiased estimator is:

$$g_i^U = c(m)g_i; \ cm \approx 1 - \frac{3}{4m - 1}$$

where m = number of degrees of freedom.

As m becomes large, g_i^U tends to g_i, so g_i is almost unbiased in large samples. Furthermore, because $c(m) < 1$, the variance of the unbiased estimator g_i^U is smaller than the variance of g_i. Therefore, g_i^U has uniformly smaller mean squared error than does g_i. In addition, Hedges has shown that this unbiased estimator has asymptotic properties.

Test of Homogeneity

Another important statistical issue that is often overlooked by meta-analysts is whether it is reasonable to assume that the population effect sizes are constant across a series of studies. Hedges (1982) cautions against making the assumption that effect sizes are constant and advises that effect sizes be tested for homogeneity. When outcome results are not homogeneous or consistent across situations, reasonable questions are raised as to the source of this variability and the subsequent justification of combining them.

Numerous tests of homogeneity are reported in the literature (Hunter et al., 1982; Gilbert, Buckman, & Mosteller, 1977; Hedges, 1982). However, the test reported by Hedges is consistent with his previous statistical considerations and is presented.

A statistical test for the homogeneity of effect size is formally a test of the hypothesis:

Ho: $£_i = £$; i = 1 . . . . . . k versus the alternative that at least one £ differs from the rest. If all the studies under review have the same population effect size (i.e., Ho is true) then the test statistic H presented by Hedges has an asymptotic chi-square distribution given by H $\sim X^2_{x-1}$. Therefore, if the obtaining value of H exceeds the $100(1-\alpha)\%$ critical value of the chi-square distribution with $(K-1)$ d.f. one would reject the hypothesis that the effects sizes are equal. The investigator may decide not to pool all the studies because they are not estimating the same parameter. Hedges found this H statistic to be slightly conservative. Also, he notes that when sample sizes are large it is probably worthwhile to consider the actual variation in the values of g_i^U because a small difference may lead to larger values of the H statistic.

Cumulation of Effect Studies

Given homogeneity of effect size, one must consider the best procedure for estimating the common effect size across studies. Most published reports calculate the average of the effect size estimates and refer to the average value as the effect size (Glass, 1976; Smith and Glass, 1977; Glass and Smith, 1977; Glass et al., 1981; Branwen, 1982). This approach is improper because there will always be bias in cumulating effect sizes across studies. Several solutions to this problem are presented in the literature.

1. One solution is to combine the studies weighing each effect size by the size of the study to derive a combined estimator (Hunter et al., 1982). One noticeable problem with this technique is that this statistic is asymptotically normally distributed only if the sample size underlying each di is large or the number of studies is large. The number of subjects and the number of different research studies is rarely large enough to warrant asymptotic theory (Hedges, 1982; Kraemer, 1983).

2. Recognizing this problem, Hedges (1982) advocates replacing di by an unbiased estimate of the population effect size. That is, one estimates the population effect size and uses the sample estimate of the population effect size to estimate the weights for each study. Hedges defines the weighted estimator by:

$$ g = \frac{\sum_{i=1}^{k} \frac{g_i^U}{\sigma_i^2(g_i^U)}}{\sum_{i=1}^{k} \frac{1}{\sigma_i^2(g_i^U)}}, $$

where $\sigma_i^2(\pounds_i)$ is given by:

$$\frac{n_i^E + n_i^C}{n_i^E n_i^C} + \frac{\delta_i^2}{2(n_i^E + n_i^C)}$$

Hedges notes that this estimate has a slight negative bias which tends to underestimate £.

3. Finally, Kraemer states that the Hedges technique is improper because the variance of di is not independent of the unknown population effect size (Kraemer, 1983). Obtaining valid confidence intervals or tests based on dw (Hedges weighted formula) under these circumstances is a problem, particularly when samples sizes are small. As a result, Kraemer advocates using the transformation:

$$r_i = d_i / (d_i^2 + 4)^{\frac{1}{2}}$$
$$Z_i = 2(n_i)$$

Analytic procedures are then applied to Z_i instead of d_i. The effect of the Kraemer transformation is to alternate size. When d_i is small, there is little change. However, when d_i is large, there is a big change. Sample size d_i has approximately a normal distribution with mean Z (p), (p = $\pounds(\pounds^2 + 4)^{\frac{1}{2}}$) and a variance equal to $(V-1)^{-1}$.

Sample Size

There are two other important issues to be considered which are discussed by only one individual in the literature (Kraemer, 1983). These two issues are disparate sample sizes for individual studies under consideration and small sample sizes for individual studies under consideration. All of the statistical evidence provided by Hedges in calculating large sample approximations of the effect size statistic has assumed equal sample sizes for both the control and experimental groups. In addition, Hedge's work has been on the assumption of $n > 20$ for each study.

Kraemer (1983) studied the effect size for studies with less than $n = 20$ and where $p = nE/N$ was $p > .4$ and $p < .6$. Looking at confidence intervals, tests of homogeneity, and the cumulation of effect sizes across studies she concluded that individual studies with less than 20 individuals and/or disparate group size are extremely problematic and should not be used.

APPLICATION OF META-ANALYSIS
IN SMALL GROUP TREATMENT RESEARCH

Small group treatment research has long been hampered by the lack of large sample sizes. One of the consequences of conducting research with small samples has been the often repeated failure to reject the null hypothesis of no differences between experimental conditions. Failing to reject the null hypothesis, researchers often abandon their present research efforts and turn their attention to new topics. This tendency is both inefficient and ineffective. The development of theoretically based treatment interventions is a cumulative endeavor. The statistical evidence gained from one experimental effort should not and can not be used to evaluate the efficacy of any treatment intervention. The efficacy of a treatment intervention can be assessed only after repeated research efforts. The statistical evidence gained from any given experiment should be used to re-define and re-shape additional long-term research efforts.

Planned statistical hypothesis testing can not be replaced by meta-analytic methods. However, meta-analysis can complement a series of long-term, developmental research efforts. In fact, it would appear that meta-analysis is well suited as a planned adjunctive statistical method.

The methodological problems associated with meta-analysis can be easily managed by the small group treatment researcher. The researcher has complete control of the independent variable and the dependent measures, the quality of the research designs, and the number of subjects per study.

The statistical evidence gained from meta-analysis can lend support for the overall efficacy of the treatment intervention. Most notably, a cumulative summary statistic of treatment effectiveness and confidence intervals for mean group difference gains can be calculated to lend support for the clinical significance of the treatment intervention.

CONCLUSION

The awareness of and application of meta-analytic methods as a means of conducting quantitative reviews of literature have greatly increased during the past decade. While techniques have much to offer, the methodological problems associated with these methods are well documented in the literature. However, the statistical problems have not been well reported in the literature. Furthermore, the use of meta-analytic procedures as an adjunctive method for long-term program development has been overlooked.

This paper has presented both the statistical problems associated with meta-analysis and the potential advantages meta-analysis has to offer for long-term program development in the area of small group treatment research. In summary, the following suggestions are provided as guidelines for the use of meta-analysis in small group treatment research.

All studies included in the meta-analysis should include both a treatment and control condition as well as appropriate randomization procedures. A minimum of twenty subjects per study is suggested. In addition, studies with disparate group sizes should be considered for exclusion from the meta-analysis. In calculating the effect size per study, use the pooled-within group standard deviation. Correct each effect size estimate using the unbiased estimator developed by Hedges. To insure that the population effect sizes are constant across the entire series of studies, select the test of homogeneity you feel is appropriate. Finally, when estimating the common effect size across all studies, cumulate the effect sizes correcting for the second level of error.

REFERENCES

Berk, A. and Chalmers, T. Costs and efficiency of the substitution of ambulatory for inpatient care. *New England Journal of Medicine,* 1981, *304*(7), 393–397.

Branwen, M. *Meta-analysis of the effectiveness of assertion training groups.* Dissertation, University of Wisconsin, 1982.

Cook, T. and Gruder, C. Meta-evaluation research. *Evaluation Quarterly,* 1978, *2,* 5–51.

Cook, T. and Leviton, L. Reviewing the literature: A comparison of traditional methods with meta-analysis. *Journal of Personality,* 1980, *48*(1), 449–472.

Cooper, H. Statistically combining independent studies: A meta-analysis of sex differences in conformity research. *Journal of Personality and Social Psychology,* 1979, *57*(1), 131–146.

Cooper, H. and Arkin, R. On quantitative reviewing. *Journal of Personality,* 1981, *49*(2), 225–229.

DeSilva, R., Henekens, C., Lewin, B., and Casscells, W. Lignocaine prophylaxis in acute myocardial infarction: An evaluation of randomized trials. *Lancet,* 1981, *2,* 855–858.

Eysenck, H. An exercise in mega-silliness. *American Psychologist,* May 1978, 517.

Gilbert, J., Buckman, M., and Mosteller, F. Progress in surgery in anesthesia: Benefits and risks of innovative therapy. In J. Bunker, B. Barnes, and F. Mosteller (Eds.), *Costs, risks, and benefits of surgery,* New York: Oxford Press, 1977, 124–145.

Glass, G. Integrating findings: The meta-analysis of research. *Review of Research in Education,* 1978, *5,* 351–379.

Glass, G. and Smith, L. Meta-analysis of research on class size and achievement. *Educational Evaluation and Policy Analysis,* 1979, *1*(1), 2–16.

Glass, G., McGraw, B., and Smith, M. *Meta-analysis in social research.* Beverly Hills, California: Sage Publishing, Inc., 1981.

Hedges, L. Distribution theory for Glass's estimator of effect size and related estimates. *Journal of Education Statistics,* 1981, *6*(2), 107–128.

Hedges, L. Estimation of effect size from a series of independent experiments. *Psychological Bulletin,* 1982, *92*(2), 490–499.

Hunter, J., Schmidt, F. and Jackson, G. *Meta-analysis: Cumulating research findings across studies.* Beverly Hills, California: Sage Publishing, Inc., 1982.

Kraemer, C. Theory of estimation of testing of effect sizes: Use in meta-analysis. *Journal of Educational Statistics,* 1983, *8*(2), 93–101.

Leviton, L. and Cook, T. What differentiates meta-analysis from other forms of review. *Journal of Personality,* 1981, *49*(2), 231–236.

Mintz, J. Integrating research evidence: A commentary on meta-analysis. *Journal of Counsulting and Clinical Psychology,* 1983, *51*(1), 71–75.

Nurius, P. Utility of data synthesis for social work. *Social Work Research and Abstracts,* 1984, *20*(3), 23–32.

Pillermer, D. and Light, R. Synthesizing outcomes: How to use research evidence from many studies. *Harvard Educational Review,* 1980, *50*(2), 176–195.

Rosenthal, R. Combining results of independent studies. *Psychological Bulletin,* 1978, *85*(1), 185–195.

Smith, M. and Glass, G. Meta-analysis of psychotherapy outcome studies. *American Psychologist,* 1977, *32,* 752–760.

Strube, M. and Hartman, D. Meta-analysis: Techniques, applications and functions. *Journal of Consulting and Clinical Psychology,* 1983, *51*(1), 14–27.

Wilson, G. and Rachman, S. Meta-analysis and the evaluation of psychotherapy outcome: Limitations and liabilities. *Journal of Consulting and Clinical Psychology,* 1983, *51*(1), 54–64.

Group Training for the Management of Chronic Pain in Interpersonal Situations

Karen Subramanian

The individual with chronic pain soon finds that all aspects of life are affected by the unrelenting physical changes experienced. Not only are major life areas of work, recreation, and family altered, but even everyday tasks such as getting dressed or performing a simple household chore may require more exertion and discomfort than the individual ever thought possible. This drastically new life pattern requires tremendous adjustment on the part of an individual. The development of new interpersonal behaviors is one major aspect of this adjustment. The need to ask for help more often, to deal with caring but overprotective family members, or to continue relationships with friends and co-workers in spite of altered circumstances all require the individual to develop new or alternative responses that will be called for many times a day.

The interpersonal contexts of patients with chronic pain are increasingly being recognized as important variables that influence the chronic pain problem itself (Turk, 1979). While recent research has indicated that psychological strategies may play an important role in reducing pain and the accompanying physical and psychosocial dysfunction (Tan, 1982; Turner & Chapman, 1982), most treatments have not focused on helping the patient adjust to the everyday interpersonal situations that arise. Instead, treatments usually consist of

Karen Subramanian, MSW, PhD, is Professor, School of Social Work, University of Southern California.

The project was carried out under the auspices of the Interpersonal Skill Training Project, School of Social Work, University of Wisconsin, Madison. This project was partially supported by funds from the Graduate School, University of Wisconsin.

55

teaching cognitive restructuring and/or relaxation skills, including the use of biofeedback. The adjustive demands confronting the individual over time are characteristics that transcend all chronic pain problems, regardless of etiology, yet relatively little attention has been afforded to effective ways of responding, meeting challenges, and restructuring lives (Turk, Sobel, Follick, & Youkilis, 1980).

This paper summarizes the interpersonal situations faced daily by persons with chronic pain. These situations were explored in a group treatment for the management of chronic pain which particularly stressed learning how to interact differently with others through the use of modeling and behavioral rehearsal of assertive techniques. This type of training has the potential to increase interpersonal effectiveness and reduce stress in daily life. Within the assertiveness area, the skills of refusals, requests, and expression of feelings were found to pertain directly to the life role changes that persons with chronic pain are undergoing. Although assertiveness has only occasionally been included in pain research studies, there are indications that it may be a valuable adjunct to other strategies in chronic pain management.

Turk et al. (1980) conceptualize coping as the effective response of the individual to specific life situations. They stress that the development of preventive or remedial programs capable of reversing maladaptive coping require detailed knowledge of the process of adaptation, a research area not yet well-developed. These authors describe a behavior-analytic approach to the process of coping which includes three tasks: problem identification, response enumeration, and response evaluation. The focus of this paper will be directed towards the first step in this three-phase approach, the need to systematically survey the problematic situations faced by individuals with a specific medical problem. In this case, the reference is to difficult interpersonal encounters faced by individuals in chronic pain. As more clinicians record and categorize these difficulties in adaptation, treatment aimed at coping with chronic pain will increasingly become more precisely targeted.

The author will begin by reviewing the relevant literature pertaining to the interpersonal context of pain. Next, the treatment program and outcome results are presented briefly.

Both the program and the results will be described in fuller detail elsewhere (Subramanian & Rose, 1985). Finally, and most important for the purpose of this paper, descriptions of the specific interpersonal situations with which the group members were struggling will be detailed.

INTERPERSONAL CONTEXT OF PAIN

Most of the research in the psychological study of chronic pain has been directed toward the evaluation of intra-individual variables. The early researchers in this area believed that operant theory could provide the basis for the necessary behavior changes. Fordyce (1976) promoted the view of pain as consisting of behaviors which are operant as well as respondent in nature. His approach involved manipulating the interpersonal consequences that are hypothesized to exert control over the continuation of patient's pain behavior. Khatami and Rush (1978) conceptualized chronic pain as having both intra- and interpersonal determinants. In addition to relaxation training or biofeedback training and cognitive therapy, their treatment used operant family therapy to effect changes in interpersonal behavior.

Heinrich, Cohen, and Naliboff (1982) have extended the study of interpersonal variables using assertiveness training. They have attempted to extend the definition and learning model of chronic pain to include interpersonal competence to effectively live day-to-day with chronic pain problems, concluding that ineffective interpersonal coping can exacerbate stress and lead to further dysfunction as well as increase the experience of pain.

Heinrich et al. (1982) found in their study of low-back pain patients that problematic interpersonal situations included the areas of health care environment, home environment, work environment, and social-recreational environment. They used assertiveness training as part of their total treatment strategy, acknowledging that this approach was largely untried for medical problems such as chronic pain. Findings showed a very positive reaction to the interpersonal skill training by patients and their spouses. The investigators concluded that " . . . such training can be successfully integrated into traditional approaches to treating pain problems and that such an integration will increase the effectiveness of the more traditional interventions and lead to increased patient satisfaction and more effective functioning" (p. 134). Their outcome study of behavioral therapy which included assertiveness training as well as relaxation and other cognitive strategies was a comparison of behavioral and physical therapy (Heinrich, Cohen, & Naliboff, 1982). Both treatments showed significant positive outcome in the areas of improved psychological and psychosocial functioning, and altered pain intensity and perception of pain.

Brooks and Richardson (1980) used assertiveness training along with anxiety management training in the treatment of eleven patients with duodenal ulcers. In comparison with eleven other patients who received an attention placebo treatment, the treatment patients reported less severe ulcer symptomatology, experienced fewer days of symptomatic pain, and consumed less antacid medication in a 60-day follow-up period. Comparison of groups 3-1/2 years later revealed a significantly lower rate of ulcer recurrence in the treatment group.

Another important benefit which may result from including modeling and behavioral rehearsal of interpersonal situations in a chronic pain management program is based on the frequent descriptions of depression as a concomitant of chronic pain (Fordyce, 1976; Sternbach, 1974). Investigators have noted similarities in cognitive and behavioral patterns among chronic pain patients and depressed individuals. These similarities include cognitive distortion, the loss of positive social reinforcement due to physical limitations and the concurrent loss of job, declining social and recreational activities, increasingly frequent cognitive appraisals of declining well-being, hopelessness regarding the future, and an inability to do anything about it (Kerns & Turk, 1984).

Empirical testing indicates the potential of using assertiveness training for the treatment of depression (Sanchez, Lewinsohn, and Larson, 1980; Comas-Diaz, 1981). Although the exact relationship of depression to chronic pain has still not been determined, there does seem to be sufficient similarity between cognitive and behavioral patterns to research the value of using behavioral treatments of depression with chronic pain patients.

THE TREATMENT PROGRAM

The pain management program described in this paper was placed within a group approach as it is believed that the use of groups in pain management will allow for an increased ability to reach many more individuals who need therapy and may enhance the effectiveness of the techniques themselves. The treatment was then compared with a waiting list control. Subjects in this study were 21 chronic pain patients (5 male and 16 female; mean age = 45). The subjects averaged 9.4 years of pain (range = 6 months to 40 years) and were a clinically varied group with causation including disease processes as well as accidents at home, on-the-job, and in motor vehicles.

Treatment consisted of ten two-hour structured group sessions which included teaching the pain management skills of relaxation training, cognitive restructuring, and social skills training. Several types of relaxation training were included, such as autogenic relaxation and imagery. Cognitive restructuring included analysis of self-enhancing/self-defeating thoughts. Assertiveness training in the areas of making requests, refusals, and expression of feeling was the primary social skill focused on within the group treatment.

Group methods included mini-lectures, discussion, and structured exercises which involved the interaction of group members, such as behavioral rehearsals. A comprehensive set of measures was obtained to assess physical and psychosocial dysfunction, mood, and pain. Information on medications and other treatments was obtained at interview sessions. Postgroup evaluations were distributed after each session in order to obtain a measure of the subjects' satisfaction with treatment and a self-report on the usefulness of treatment.

Results indicated that the treatment group improved significantly on measures of physical and psychosocial functioning and negative mood states from pre- to post-test while the control group had virtually no change or worsened. There were statistically significant differences in gains between the control and treatment groups at post-test, and these gains were also judged to be clinically important results. Four-month follow-up results demonstrated that the significant physical and psychosocial improvements were maintained.

Although negative mood states were still reduced from pre-test, they were no longer significant. Measures of pain indicated small reductions from pre to post for both treatment and control, although the treatment group had significant pain reductions at follow-up.

Post and follow-up interviews with subjects indicated that subjects developed an increased sense of self-acceptance from the treatment. Apparently, many subjects enter treatment believing that since they can no longer perform in the roles they had filled previous to their pain condition, they are now devalued as people—not as good or as useful as they used to be. The treatment process results in their being more accepting of who they are now and what roles there are still left for them to fill. Members reported that the mutual support of the group was very important to them.

PROBLEM IDENTIFICATION
OF INTERPERSONAL CONTEXTS

In order to develop knowledge about the problems that chronic pain patients have in daily interpersonal contexts, an analysis was made of all such situations that members brought to the group. Information was derived from three sources. First, a tally was made of situations described in members' weekly written home assignments. These home assignments included describing how members had attempted to apply their newly learned coping skills to actual situations they encountered during the week. Second, each leader made post-group notes of significant problems verbalized by members in each group session. Third, the presenting problem situations mentioned by members in the pre-group interviews were added to the tally. The resulting total of 69 difficult interpersonal situations were placed within the four categories of Heinrich et al. (1982) in order to generalize the usefulness of these findings and add additional content validity to the categories themselves. These four categories were: social/recreational environment, home environment, work environment, and health environment (see table opposite).

Tally of Interpersonal Situations Presented
by Group Members

Category	Number of Situations Tallied	Percentage of Total Situations
Social/Recreational	17	25%
Home	35	51%
Work	14	20%
Health Care	3	4%
Total	69	100%

Although behavioral interactions are always accompanied by cognitive processes, these latter processes will not be explored in this paper in order to focus on the relatively more explored area of interpersonal interactions. In treatment, however, cognitive and behavioral work go hand in hand. The description of these interpersonal situations and suggestions for treatment follows.

Social/Recreational Environment

Most chronic pain conditions are not present at birth. They occur to individuals at some point in their lives, presenting themselves as the result of accidents, development of disease, deterioration of body functioning, and so forth. This new and traumatic situation forces an individual and the surrounding support group to adapt to a new way of life. If adaptation is unsatisfactory, the support group will diminish contact with the patient, resulting at times in divorce or the loss of friends. This loss of contact with people is often not remedied by the introduction of new social supports because the presence of chronic pain inhibits a person from going out and making new contacts. Group members described a total of 17 situations (24%) in which they had difficulty in the social and recreational environment.

It was found that group members cut off potential social or

recreational activities because they have special needs that they do not wish to impose on others. For example, group members have declined to go to the movies with friends because lengthy sitting would be painful, declined a social visit because climbing the stairs would be too difficult, or declined a Sunday drive in the country because the car ride would be uncomfortable and not worth the effort.

When group members do decide to involve themselves in a social activity, they sometimes find that the pain becomes so intense that it interferes with their enjoyment. However, members have often chosen to try and endure their discomfort rather than disrupt the activity. When this behavior is analyzed more closely, several possible explanations arise. One reason is that some individuals believe that responding to pain by changing a behavior (such as leaving a party) is equated with allowing pain to rule their lives. Secondly, an unwillingness on the part of some people to display dependence and/or impose their disability on others is common. For example, group members frequently found that their need to ask for an early ride home from a particular event consequently ended the activity for others as well; thus, they resisted going home early.

Friends or neighbors sometimes make requests of group members that are liable to increase physical discomfort and fatigue. Saying "no" at these times was frequently a difficult task for members. For example, a neighbor would ask for a favor such as shopping or babysitting, not realizing the extent of the member's disability. When the severity of the disability varies from day to day, non-intimate social contacts may not realize that a member who is active one day may be much more disabled with pain the next day. Another type of situation occurs when members do not work because of their pain conditions and are at home during the day. Friends may come to visit and not realize that their stay is overlong and fatiguing. Individuals with chronic pain face a dual problem in learning to cope effectively with these situations. First, in order to admit disability to another person one must first be able to accept that disability within oneself (a cognitive problem). Secondly, coping in these situations may require the use of assertiveness skills in areas of life never needed before.

Assertiveness training as part of a total pain management

program has the potential to teach these individuals more effective coping skills with the goal of reducing social isolation resulting from disability. Examples may be drawn from the treatment group described in this paper. Members practiced telling their friends that they would really enjoy a Sunday car ride, and then asking if the ride could have some rest stops built into the plan. Before going to a movie with friends, a member requested arriving early so that she could obtain the aisle seat, thus allowing unobtrusive stretching whenever needed. When stairs were impossible to climb, another member practiced requesting an alternate meeting place rather than cancel the appointment. Other assertive practice was directed to saying "no" politely but firmly to requests by friends and neighbors, with the member choosing whether or not the disability was to be given as the reason for refusal. Members found that as it became easier to say "no" when they needed to, their social interactions were enhanced. When they were able to help others, they did it freely and not because they felt coerced. Members also avoided people less, as avoidance was a coping method used previously to defend against unwanted requests.

Home Environment

It is often difficult for family members to understand the changed physical and mental state of the person who develops a condition of chronic pain, resulting in unsatisfactory adaptation and communication. In the family's attempts to help, they may seek to remove excess pressure and responsibility from the individual. For example, they might begin to urge physician's visits, medications, appropriate activities, etc. They might also take over the person's daily tasks or finish tasks that seem to take a longer time than previously. If these changes occur without the active involvement and agreement of the disabled individual, they may be seen by that individual as a statement of inability to function or to make decisions, resulting in resentment and further interference with communication. Family members may not realize, for example, that although a task may get done more slowly, the individual needs to finish the work to maintain self-esteem.

Group members found that they needed help and support

from their family more than ever before, yet they also continually struggled to retain their functioning roles within the family, thus indicating the need to learn a delicate balance between dependence and independence. Some male group members, who had previously held traditional roles within their families, have had to switch or share roles with their wives. They struggle with personal adjustment issues resulting from losing their role as breadwinner or having to now share the role of the "strong one" in the family. Group members identified 35 (51%) situations in which they had interpersonal difficulties in the home environment, indicating that this was the most problematic area of the four being presented.

Many members cannot perform the household responsibilities that they did formerly; this sometimes has resulted in feelings of helplessness and uselessness. If sexual activity has also diminished, the feelings of uselessness only increase. Members sometimes identified themselves as burdens to their families. When members must reduce the physical tasks that they perform around the home, they often harbor guilt feelings about not doing their "fair share." This feeling of guilt compounds the situation when a member, in attempting to perform a task, finds it necessary to ask for assistance. Thus, members may persist at completing a task even if it results in increased physical discomfort. Some members feel this struggle for maintenance of their family role so keenly that they may persist alone in a task until the increased pain is so intense that it requires bedrest.

Women members who were raised with traditional social and religious values that emphasized always thinking of others before themselves felt very uncomfortable about making requests or asking for special privileges, even when demanded by a condition of chronic pain. For example, they believed that it was selfish of them to ask others to help fulfill the homemaker role that was their responsibility, yet they had enormous difficulty continuing to fulfill the demands of the role all alone, thus resulting in a continuing inner struggle that occasionally reflected itself in outbursts to the family.

Some members were forced to decrease their physical interaction with their children because of pain, creating another source of guilt. This proved to be especially true for traditionally raised men who saw themselves as role models for their male children in the areas of sports and physically hard work. The primary relationship these men had held with their children was based on physical activity, and other potential areas of relationship (such as quiet companionship, reading) were both underdeveloped and devalued.

A major aim of treatment in the area of Home Environment consisted of helping members to accept themselves in new family roles, new roles that were as essential and important to family functioning as the old roles had appeared to be. Assertiveness training along with cognitive restructuring is useful in helping members begin to behaviorally enact and try out these new roles. Through trying out new patterns of behavior, members can begin to view themselves as whole individuals with new roles in the family and to understand that they can still be useful and productive members of their families. Although it is a gradual process, group members begin to realize that their value does not lie in the number of tasks they accomplish, but in how they interact and communicate with family members.

As new roles are discussed cognitively in the group, assertive statements become the vehicle for changing roles. For example, a father whose small children were used to playing rough and tumble games with him before his accident, had only been able to respond to the children by saying that he could not play. The children would go away confused and he would isolate himself, feeling saddened and useless. During the group treatment, this individual was able to practice statements that could help him develop a new basis for relating to his children. For example, saying: "No, boys, I can't play ball with you today because my back is hurting. How about when you're through playing, I'll read you a story (take a walk with you, etc.)?"

Work Environment

Of the ten group members, three were unable to work because of their pain condition. For some individuals, giving up employment because of disability is the greatest adjustment of all and may be reflected in lowered self-esteem. Seven group members were either working part-time or attending college. In either of these situations, the indivdiuals were having to adapt to the demands of a work environment which required a certain level of productivity, usually within a limited time frame. There were 14 situations (20%) described by these latter group members with reference to difficulties in their work or school situations.

For members who attempted to return to full-time employment after the development of their pain condition, they found that fatigue and pain became too intense to complete a regular work day. These members adapted by reducing their work hours to a part-time basis. Problems faced by members at work included having to sit for long periods of time at meetings, not being able to meet deadlines because of unexpected exacerbations of their physical condition, and not being able to stand or work as much as the job demanded. One salesman with a back and leg problem was hindered from his work because he had great difficulty getting in and out of a car all day. This individual eventually gave up his job completely.

Group members who were working were particularly sensitive about appearing "normal" in front of co-workers, and in certain situations, customers. Difficulties often arose as they experienced pain during the normal workday and tried to hide it. The members feared that if they showed their pain, they would be seen as less productive, resulting in reduced confidence on the part of their employers and possibly the loss of their jobs.

One of the potential applications of assertiveness training in the Work Environment is to help members learn to express their special needs on-the-job. A few members who did practice and eventually express their special needs to co-workers, such as rearranging furniture for easier reaching or requesting a special chair, found co-workers to be agreeable. These small but important changes increased the members' productivity and certainly their attitude on the job.

Health Environment

Although Heinrich et al. (1980) cite Health Care Environment as a demanding one for pain patients, group members had only three situations in this category (4%). Problems listed by Heinrich et al. include patients being confronted with examinations and treatment procedures that they do not understand, yet being afraid to question their physicians. In addition, there may be problematic encounters with other health care providers such as physical therapists, social workers, secretaries, nurses, etc. Often patients are unsure as to why they are meeting with various professionals and feel uncomfortable displaying their lack of understanding.

The three group members who did have difficult interpersonal encounters with health care professionals cited the following concerns. One member felt that she was treated impersonally and rudely during her tests, yet she did not know how to react in this situation. A second member found her physician giving her very little information during her visit, but had a fear of asking the physician questions. Another group member, who had four hip replacements in eight years, finds it now difficult to trust any physician. As a result, he may not seek medical care when it is necessary.

CONCLUSIONS

Although the interpersonal context of pain is increasingly being recognized as an important factor in satisfactory life adjustment, few research or treatment programs focus on the remediation of unsatisfactory relationships. One of the first steps in remedying this treatment gap is interpersonal problem identification. This paper has sought to make more explicit the specific types of interpersonal problems which confront individuals living with chronic pain. A study of the particular situations with which people are struggling can give clearer ideas of what people need in treatment.

The author has described a group treatment program which seeks to directly impact the manner in which these individuals respond to their interpersonal environment. The results of this treatment program which emphasized modeling and behavioral rehearsal present additional evidence that cognitive and behavioral interventions are effective in reducing dysfunction in subjects with chronic pain. Although these results must be regarded tentatively because of the small sample size in this study, it does appear that group treatment of this type has the potential to increase the coping skills of persons living with chronic pain.

Despite the presence of conditions that are clearly traumatic and disruptive, many persons with chronic pain are able to make satisfactory adjustments to their lives. This indicates that in addition to pain, social and cognitive factors determine the degree of satisfactory adaptation. The teaching of new and alternative interpersonal responses can assist these individuals to cope as they face the daily tasks of living.

REFERENCES

Bergner, M., Bobbitt, R.A., & Pollard, W.E., "The Sickness Impact Profile: Validation of a Health Status Measure," *Medical Care,* 1976, *14,* 56.

Brooks, Gary R., & Richardson, Frank C., "Emotional Skills Training: A Treatment Program for Duodenal Ulcer," *Behavior Therapy,* 1980, *11,* 198–207.

Comas-Diaz, Lillian, "Effects of Cognitive and Behavioral Group Treatment on the Depressive Symptomatology of Puerto Rican Women," *Journal of Consulting and Clinical Psychology,* 1981, *49*(5), 627–632.

Fordyce, Wilbert E., *Behavioral Methods for Chronic Pain and Illness,* St. Louis: C.V. Mosby Co., 1976.

Heinrich, Richard L., Cohen, Michael J., & Naliboff, Bruce D., "Rehabilitation of Pain Patients: Coping in Interpersonal Contexts," in Joseph Barber and Cheri Adrian, (Eds.), *Psychological Approaches to the Management of Pain,* New York: Brunner/Mazel, 1982.

Kerns, R.D. & Turk, D.C., "Depression and Chronic Pain: The Mediating Role of the Spouse," *Journal of Marriage and The Family,* 1984, 845–852.

Khatami, Manoochehr, and Rush, A. John, "A Pilot Study of the Treatment of Outpatients with Chronic Pain: Symptom Control, Stimulus Control and Social System Intervention," *Pain,* 1978, *5,* 163–172.

McNair, D.M., Lorr, M., and Droppleman, L.F., *Profile of Mood States,* San Diego, Ca.: Educational and Industrial Testing Service, 1971.

Metcalfe, M., & Goldman, E., "Validation of an Inventory for Measuring Depression," *British Journal of Psychiatry,* 1965, *111,* 241–242.

Novaco, Raymond W., "Anger and Coping with Stress," in John P. Foreyt and Diana P. Rathjen (Eds.), *Cognitive Behavior Therapy: Research and Application,* New York: Plenum Press, 1978.

Sanchez, Victor C., Lewinsohn, Peter M., & Larson, Douglas W., "Assertion Training: Effectiveness in the Treatment of Depression," *Journal of Clinical Psychology,* 1980, *36* (2), 526–529.

Sternbach, R.S., *Pain Patients: Traits and Treatment,* New York: Academic Press, 1974.

Subramanian, Karen & Rose, Sheldon D., "Group Treatment for the Management of Chronic Pain," *Social Work Research and Abstracts Research Note, 21,* Fall 1985, 29–30.

Tan, Siang-Yang, "Cognitive and Cognitive-Behavioral Methods for Pain Control: A Selective Review," *Pain,* 1982, *12,* 201–228.

Turk, Dennis, Sobel, Harry J., Follick, Michael J., & Youkilis, Hildreth D., "A

Sequential Criterion Analysis for Assessing Coping with Chronic Illness," *Journal of Human Stress,* June, 1980, 35–40.

Turk, Dennis C., "Factors Influencing the Adaptive Process with Chronic Illness: Implications for Intervention," in G. Sarason & C.D. Speilberger (Eds.), *Stress and Anxiety,* (vol.7), Washington, D.C.: Halsted Press, 1979.

Turner, Judith A., and Chapman, Richard C., "Psychological Interventions for Chronic Pain: A Critical Review. II. Operant Conditioning, Hypnosis, and Cognitive-Behavioral Therapy," *Pain,* 1982, *12,* 23–40.

A Multimethod Group Approach: Program Development Research

Sheldon D. Rose
Steven H. Tallant
Richard Tolman
Karen Subramanian

In spite of the concern for accountability in social work practice for the past ten years, and the commitment to empiricism in some corners of the social work profession, few systematic research programs for the evaluation of social work methods have been developed. Even examples of isolated research projects evaluating practice are difficult to find. The purpose of this paper is to present the results and process to date of a comprehensive research development program of a multimethod group approach to the treatment of a wide variety of stress related presenting problems. Although this program has been in operation for five years (See Tolman and Rose, 1985), it is still in progress. During this period the program has been proposed, altered, tried out, experimented with, adjusted, and expanded to a wide variety of presenting problems. A number of products, too, have been realized. In this paper the structure of this program, its products, the process, its problems, future perspectives, and the research outcomes will be summarized.

This program has been characterized by a central theme, development and evaluation of a multimethod group ap-

Sheldon D. Rose is Professor, School of Social Work, University of Wisconsin, Madison, Wisconsin. Captain Steven H. Tallant is Director, Alcoholism Rehabilitation Center, USAF Medical Center, Scott, AFB, Illinois. Richard Tolman is with the School of Social Service Administration, University of Chicago, Chicago, Illinois. Karen Subramanian is Professor, School of Social Work, University of Southern California, Los Angeles, California.

Support for the research in all of the projects reported in this paper was provided in part by the Research funds of the Graduate School of the University of Wisconsin-Madison.

71

proach with typical client populations for commonly occurring client complaints. The structure of this program has been a series of small experimental control group projects each of which builds on the previous projects. The experiments in each project have been preceded by a review of the literature, the development of a specific protocol, the development of a detailed leader's guide based on that protocol, the evaluation and selection of a number of research instruments appropriate to the specific project, the training of leaders, and a series of data-based case studies. The latter are before-after studies without a control group. In both case studies and experiments, group process data were gathered from a weekly post session questionnaire for all clients, the results of a simple observation schedule, and such information as assignment completion and attendance (see Rose, 1984, for details on these group related instruments).

The project leader in each study had to build substantial community contacts in order to recruit a sufficient number of clients. These contacts were not only with social agencies but also with the media. As a result each project grew slowly; it usually took three years from the beginning of each project to the writing of the final report. Many of the projects reported here are interrelated and draw upon the community relations established in previous projects.

The project leaders in most cases have been advanced PhD students interested in clinical research. The group leaders had been former MSW students who had earlier received at least a part of their trianing within the program and who had led at least one group but in most cases many prior to the experiment. In no cases did the experiments themselves involve inexperienced students for leaders, although closely supervised students were used in the data-based case studies. Before the specific projects are described, a brief overview of the multimethod group approach as it has thus far developed will provide a greater understanding of the separate projects.

THE MULTIMETHOD GROUP APPROACH

Since this method is described in detail elsewhere (Rose and Edleson, 1986; Tolman and Rose, 1985) only a brief summary of the approach will be provided here. The major characteristics of the approach are the following. First, in addition to being the context of change, the group is the source of major intervention strategies designed to mediate individual learning and change. Second, the focus of treatment is on the development of coping strategies for dealing with specific problem situations. Clients are trained in a variety of coping strategies such as assertion, systematic problem solving, cognitive restructuring, relaxation and the decision-making process of how to select and apply these and other strategies when appropriate. Clients are taught how to spell out situations in such a way as to point to the coping strategies required to deal with them.

The approach is carried out in such a way as to gradually increase maximum participation and involvement in goal setting, planning, decision-making, and mutual helping of others. The process moves from high leader-given structure to low leader-given structure. Although meetings have structured agendas (see Rose, Tolman, and Tallant, 1985, for a list of these agendas) which are usually followed, the agendas serve as a point of departure for the members in the later sessions.

Another guiding principle, often difficult to achieve in groups, is maximum individualization. Each client is helped to establish individualized problem situations, goals, and coping skills. Overlapping of client situations and goals in any one group occurs in so far as each group has a common theme, e.g., stress management, pain management, anger control, depression. In developing coping strategies, effort is made to draw upon the personal resources of the clients, skills they already have, knowledge already accrued to help themselves and their fellow members. This is another way to individualize the treatment without losing the benefit of the group.

Change or maintenance of change in the specific areas mentioned above is not enough. The ultimate focus is on the transfer and maintenance of change beyond the boundaries of the group. Incorporated into every agenda, but especially in later agendas, is preparation for generalization.

Finally, the approach is characterized by the use of data in assessing the specific focus of treatment, making clinical decisions, examining the ongoing group process, and evaluating outcomes. It is this characteristic that so readily lends the approach to the possibility of systematic evaluation and research.

The characteristics of the approach that link it to traditional social work values and general social work approaches are its emphasis first on individualization and maximum involvement of members. Second, the focus is on extragroup or environmental means of intervention when group and individual interventions are not sufficient and on the skills of the group worker in establishing effective working relationships with the clients. Third, the dignity of the individual is maintained throughout treatment by making the client aware of all techniques to be used prior to their application and then only with the consent of the client. In addition, the approach is primarily positive in nature with a great deal of support for the ongoing efforts of the clients.

Because the method uses a wide variety of group procedures to increase the attraction of the group to its members, ensure broad participation, set limits on deviant members, resolve group problems, establish pro-therapeutic group norms, and enhance the mutual helping effect of its members, it must draw heavily upon group theory, group dynamics research (Cartwright and Zander, 1968), and traditional group work practice (e.g., Heap, 1984).

The cognitive-behavioral paradigm emphasizes the use of data, specific problem formulation, the use of such procedures as cognitive restructuring, assertive training, relaxation, reinforcement, and the inclusion of generalization strategies. For this reason the multimethod approach also draws heavily on cognitive-behavioral theory and the work of Bandura (1971) and Meichenbaum (1977) in particular. It is our contention that these various theoretical traditions and paradigms are not incompatible. To the contrary, they supplement each other to provide the most effective treatment to the client. Let us examine the specific projects around which this developmental research program has been organized. The first is the treatment of chronic stress.

CHRONIC STRESS

Clients suffering from chronic stress were selected as the target of the first project in which to evaluate a multimethod approach because the diversity of the manifestations of chronic stress seemed to require a broad-based and diverse treatment program. Furthermore, in learning to deal with stressful situations more effectively, clients should generally improve their capacity to deal with a wide range of stress and anxiety-related problems. In individual therapy, similar though less broad-based programs have been used to treat problems of pain management and anger control. Somewhat modified versions have been used in the treatment of depression both individually and in groups.

We selected a stress management package because of its compatibility with a group approach and because of the large number of clients in the community who complained of stress as one of their major problems. The many exercises used in stress management readily lend themselves to mutual problem solving, group support, peer interaction procedures, and other group procedures. As a result the group should supplement the structured program and increase its effectiveness. Another reason to select clients with chronic stress as the initial target was that since stress is a subjective experience, the use of self-reports could be used to evaluate outcomes of stress treatment studies.

Several of the ingredients of a multimethod approach include group methods, relational methods, extragroup methods, and assertion training—a package with which we have had extensive clinical experience and positive research results. Thus, we selected the stress management program because we could build on our earlier research program (for example, Schinke and Rose, 1976; Toseland and Rose, 1978) by adding primarily cognitive procedures, and relaxation training to an already familiar approach. Moreover, we could maintain many of our community agency contacts.

Finally, we could draw upon five research studies in which stress management was taught using some, but not all of the ingredients of a multimethod group package and which had a control group (Forman, 1982; Decker, Williams, and Hall, 1982; Sarason, Johnson, Berberich, and Siegel, 1979; Kelly, Bradlyn, Dubbert, and St. Lawrence, 1982; Tisdelle, Hansen, St. Lawrence, Kelly, and Brown, 1983). Only one of the five studies reported no significant differences between the stress management condition and a wait-list condition at either posttest or at follow-up (Sarason et al., 1979). All of the other studies report significant differences on a variety of dependent measures ranging from physiological to self-report measures. For the most part, these studies all have methodological weaknesses (i.e., use of intact groups and lack of random assignment). Despite their limitations these studies still lend modest support for the overall effectiveness of stress management techniques on a variety of dependent measures.

For this reason the further development of the multimethod group approach seemed at a minimum to require further research in which methodological errors of the earlier studies were corrected and the entire multimethod group package was utilized. Such a study was designed by Tolman and Rose (1985).

STRESS MANAGEMENT AND RELAXATION TRAINING IN GROUPS

In order to test the package which was theoretically derived from the various paradigms mentioned, four groups over a two-year period were organized and run for eight weeks. Two were sponsored by the Interpersonal Skill Training and Research Project of the School of Social Work and two others by a private family service agency. Most clients who completed the program showed major changes on the outcome measures indicating a self-reported decrease in stress. However, in the absence of a control group a number of alternative explanations could not be run.

For this reason the Tolman-Rose (1985) study compared the multimethod stress management package (SP) with a relaxation only (RO) comparison condition and a wait-list (WL) condition. Forty-five subjects were randomly assigned to the various conditions. The use of appropriate randomization procedures was a noted improvement compared to previous stress management studies which generally failed to randomize subjects. Randomization resulted in a total of 13 subjects assigned to the stress management condition, 14 subjects assigned to the relaxation only condition, and 13 subjects assigned to the wait-list. The subjects in the experimental and relaxation condition were assigned to one of two groups. Experienced leaders were also randomly assigned to one group in each condition.

Subjects in both treatment conditions participated in a total of eight two-hour weekly group sessions. Post-test evaluations were administered following the completion of the final group session. A three-month follow-up was conducted for treatment subjects. The major tests used were the Profile of Mood States (POMS), the Daily Hassles Scales, and the SCL-90-R. In addition, a self-monitoring procedure was used in which clients monitored their own levels of stress (on a 1–10 scale) three times per day.

The Profile of Mood States (POMS) (McNair, Lorr, and Droppelman, 1971, provide a test manual) is designed to measure subjective reports of affect and mood. It consists of a 65-item, 5 point rating scale for the following affective states: Tension-Anxiety, Depression-Dejection, Anger-Hostility, Vigor-Activity, Fatigue-Inertia, Confusion-Bewilderment. A total mood disturbance score (POMSTOT) is also obtainable, and was the primary score used in all of the following studies.

The Daily Hassles Scale, described by Kanner, Coyne, Schaeffer, and Lazarus (1981), consists of 117 items which sample hassles from work, family, friends, the environment, practical considerations, and chance occurrences. Because the theoretical and procedural framework of the stress management package focuses on subjects' perceived hassles, or stressors, the Hassles Scale provides a measure with high utility. The test provides a "frequency of hassles" score and a "severity of hassles" score.

The SCL-90-R is an inventory measuring symptomatic psychological distress on nine symptom dimensions: Somatization, obsessive-compulsiveness, interpersonal sensitivity, depression, anxiety, hostility, phobic anxiety, paranoid ideation, and psychoticism. The General Severity Index (GSI), which yields a score of combined symptom number and intensity, was the primary measure used (see, Derogatis, 1977), for details of the test).

Non-parametric procedures were used to analyze the data on four primary dependent measures of stress: SCL-90-R; Profile of Mood States; Self-Monitoring; and Daily Hassles Scale. At post-test, non-parametric ANCOVA analysis revealed no significant differences among the multimethod, re-

laxation only, or waiting-list control on the five measures of
stress. At the three-month follow-up there were no significant differences between the two experimental conditions.
No follow-up was carried out for the control group who
received the multimethod group program during that three-
month period. Within-group analysis showed that both the
multimethod and the relaxation programs had significant
pre- to post-test improvement whereas the untreated controls
did not show significant improvement although they indeed
showed some improvement. In the absence of significant differences between control and experimental and between experimental groups, this study did not lend support to the
efficacy of a multimethod approach. However, the size of
the treatment effect in the clinical groups and several methodological errors detected in later analysis warranted at
least replication of the research.

Moreover, the results of the Wilcoxon tests revealed, for
the most part, that the treatment conditions were successful in
bringing about improvements in stress measures from pre-
treatment baseline levels. The wait-list controls did not con-
sistently show such improvements.

Furthermore, the stress management package was *consis-
tently* superior to the wait-list control on all measures while
the relaxation condition was superior only on some of the
measures. Despite the lack of statistical significance the consistent pattern of superiority offers some evidence that the
treatment might be effective in reducing stress.

Finally, when one examines the level of improvement in
both treatment groups one can argue that the improvements
are at least clinically significant. For example, the GSI Index
of the SCL-90-R revealed that subjects at pre-test were for
the most part at distressed levels. Following treatment, both
treatment conditions had reduced their levels of symptomatology by a standard deviation bringing the subjects within normal levels of stress. The evidence suggests that the treatment
intervention was clinically significant in that treatment was
able to bring about important behavioral change. (Tables
showing the exact data are to be found in Tolman and Rose,
1984, or on request from the second author.)

While the statistical results indicated that the current
treatment package was unable to result in rejection of the

null hypothesis, the clinical trends suggested another conclusion. Since the evidence was mixed it would have been difficult at that time to regard the current package as ineffective and to develop a new treatment program. It appeared more reasonable to examine possible hypotheses which could explain the non-statistical results and from this examination to conduct a new study to evaluate the effectiveness of the current stress management package. After detailed analysis, it was concluded that a new study should be altered in the following ways:

1. Increase the power of the statistical tests by either increasing sample size or reducing the number of comparison conditions;
2. While keeping the same treatment components, increase the effectiveness of treatment by refining the treatment techniques;
3. Limit the number of students selected as subjects to only those who manifest clinical levels of stress. In the original study a number of students entered the program with low levels of reported stress;
4. Delay the post-test assessment until after the Christmas holiday period, since before that period we noted in our non-experimental groups an overall reduction of stress in all populations whether or not treatment occurred. This was not typical of other periods;
5. Control for social support as a mediating variable; theory suggests that this may be an intervening variable.

STRESS MANAGEMENT AND SOCIAL SUPPORT

The purpose of the second study was twofold: First, to continue to evaluate the treatment effectiveness of a multi-method group approach in the treatment of stress management; second, to examine the role of social support as a significant external factor in reducing stress symptomatology.

Based upon transactional stress and group treatment theory, treatment components included teaching the cognitive-behavioral skills of relaxation, cognitive-restructuring and assertiveness within a structured small group setting. In this study we corrected for the potential errors noted in the previous study. It was again hypothesized that subjects receiving group treatment would obtain significantly greater decreases in stress than subjects in a waiting-list condition. In addition, combining transactional stress and social support theory, it was hypothesized that wait-list subjects with high levels of social support would exhibit significantly greater decreases in stress than wait-list subjects with low levels of social support.

To investigate the hypotheses, a matched-pair randomized block design was utilized. Thirty-two subjects (8 male and 24 female; mean age 38), a clinical population, were rank-ordered on a measure of perceived social support, matched according to level of social support, and randomized into either treatment or wait-list condition. Treatment consisted of eight two-hour weekly group sessions using the multimethod group approach.

The statistical and clinical results described lend support to the contribution of the stress management package in reducing stress when compared to no treatment intervention. On all dependent measures of stress the treatment subjects evidenced significant pre-posttest reductions. Furthermore, on three of the four measures the treatment subjects evidenced significant pre-posttest reductions in stress compared to the wait-list subjects. Clinically, most clients moved from pathological to non-pathological categories on most of the dependent measures.

Statistical analysis failed to reveal support for hypothesis two. There were no significant differences between wait-list subjects with high social support and low social support. In fact, the analysis indicated the low social support subjects improved markedly when compared to the high social support subjects. These results suggest that the assumed benefits derived from high levels of social support are negligible and, in fact, may increase in many instances the perception of stress. (For details of these data see Tallant, Rose, and Tolman, 1985, or on request from the second author.)

Based on the results of the second study, one can assume that the multimethod group approach is more effective than a wait-list measurement-only condition in increasing the capacity of clients to cope with stress. We do not have evidence that it is better than any specified active alternative as yet, although nowhere in the literature have we found such strong treatment effects. We are also confident that in spite of the differences between the two studies, since the second corrected for methodological errors, its results should be considered the more relevant.

GROUP VERSUS INDIVIDUAL STRESS MANAGEMENT

In a third project, in order to examine the contribution of the group element in treatment, we compared the use of group and individual multimethod packages (Rose, Tallant, and Lee, 1985). Twenty subjects (16 females and 4 males, ages 19 to 47), recruited through posters and newspaper ads, were assigned randomly to one of two conditions. There were 10 subjects in the group condition and 8 individual clients, as one subject in the individual condition was referred elsewhere for a serious psychological disturbance which was unrelated to the theme of the group. A second person in the individual condition dropped out. The subjects in the group condition were randomly assigned to each group. Each group met for eight weeks with one experienced leader. Individual treatment consisted of eight one-hour sessions. The same two social workers were used for both group and individual treatment. The same program was followed as far as the therapeutic context permitted. There were six clients in each group. (As the reader will note, the number of subjects were extremely small because of difficulty in recruiting more subjects at that time.)

Clients in the group condition showed significant shifts as tested by a two-sample matched pairs Wilcoxon from pre- to post-tests on the Daily Hassles Scale (p < .05). The clients in the individual treatment condition showed significant shifts on the Hassles. Neither showed significant shifts on the POMS. There were no drop-outs in the group treatment condition but there were two drop-outs in the individual treatment condition. The clients in both conditions reported that they were extremely pleased with the kind of treatment they received and were glad that they were not in the alternate condition. Although gains in the group were somewhat larger than those in the individual treatment, there were no significant differences between the two groups. Because of the small N and the predicted likelihood of small differences in treatment effects, and the use of a two-tailed test, in retrospect we concluded that the lack of power made it unlikely that we could reject the null hypotheses. However, the fact that the cost of treatment was dramatically less for the group condition was for the moment sufficient evidence to suggest that further investigation in this area would be fruitful with a larger N, a one-tailed test, and a control on leader cost all of which would increase the power of the testing. (Complete data are to be found in Rose, Tallant, and Lee, 1985, or on request from the first author.)

PAIN MANAGEMENT

Millions of Americans suffer from chronic pain that cannot be adequately controlled. These patients spend thousands of dollars each year seeking treatment to relieve their pain, which is often made worse through medications that lead to narcotic addiction and multiple surgeries that may not be successful. Recent research has indicated that psychological strategies may in many cases play an important role in reducing pain and the accompanying physical and psychosocial dysfunction. Five of these strategies were combined into a structured group approach in order to examine their effectiveness for the management of chronic pain (Subramanian and Rose, 1985). Strategies used in treatment included relaxation training to reduce muscle tension which may increase the experience of pain, cognitive restructuring to change negative and self-defeating thoughts and feelings about the pain, social skills training to increase interpersonal effectiveness and reduce stress in daily life, group procedures to enhance participation and cohesion of the group, and relational skills to establish and maintain the attraction of the leader. These procedures were utilized within the context of a group.

The first step of the project included leader training, development of a leader's manual with agendas, mini-lectures, and exercises (Rose and Subramanian, 1985), and liaison work with hospitals and clinics in the university and community setting. The second stage included a pilot study which resulted in data on twelve subjects from three pain groups. Physical and psychosocial dysfunction as well as negative mood states decreased at post-test and again at follow-up. Pre- to follow-up improvement of subjects was significant. Findings indicated that the actual experience of pain was not affected by treatment at post-test and follow-up.

The experimental study hypothesized that the multimethod group approach would be more effective than a wait-list control in reducing physical and psychosocial dysfunction as measured by the Sickness Impact Profile and in reducing negative mood states as measured by the Profile of Mood States. It was also predicted that the gains made by the treatment group would be significantly higher than those made by the control group. Subjects in this study were 21 chronic pain patients (5 male and 16 female; mean age = 45) referred from physicians and self-referred. The subjects averaged 9.4 years of pain (range = 6 months to 40 years) and were a clinically varied group with causation including disease processes as well as accidents at home, on-the-job, and in motor vehicles. Various outcome measures as well as measures of the pain experience were completed by subjects at pre-treatment and at post-treatment. Follow-up took place three months after the end of treatment.

Subjects were initially assigned randomly to treatment and control. Because of recruitment difficulties, additional subjects were added to the control group within the first month after treatment began in order to form the sample of 21. This equivalent control group (n = 10) was similar when compared on demographics and pre-test scores on the major dependent variables.

Although measures of the pain experience indicated no change from pre- to post-test for either treatment or control, results for the major dependent variable measuring physical and phychosocial dysfunction (Sickness Impact Profile) indicated that the treatment group improved significantly from pre- to post-test while the control group had virtually no change. Results for the measure of negative mood states (Profile of Mood States) indicated that the control group worsened over time while the treatment group again made significant improvement. Both of these measures showed statistically significant differences in gains between the control and treatment groups. Although results must be regarded tentatively because of the small sample size, it does appear that the multimethod group treatment approach has the potential to increase the coping skills of persons living with chronic pain. Future studies are presently aimed at replicating the study with a randomized, and control group design. Stress and pain have not been the only targets of the multimethod group approach. (For a complete detail of data, see Subramanian and Rose, 1985, or on request from the second author.) A completely different target population, spouse abusers, has also been the client population in a series of multimethod groups. Although the experimental phase has not yet been completed, the plan has been included here to show the scope within which a multimethod group approach is being considered.

SPOUSE ABUSE

Spouse abuse, once thought to be a rare phenomenon, has emerged as a serious and widespread problem. Although there are many approaches to the treatment of the problem, at least two are concerned with the behavior of the batterer. One of these is a multimethod group program which teaches alternative responses to stressful situations previously associated with violent responses. Another is a self-help approach, Batterers Anonymous, which focuses on attitudinal revision. The purpose of this project is to examine the efficacy of both approaches and the patients each serves most effectively in terms of seriousness of the offense, duration, age, alternate therapies received, education, and socioeconomic variables.

A number of data-based case studies have been carried out by Saunders and Hanusa (1982), Edleson, (1984) and Edleson, Miller, Stone, and Chapman (1985) with positive results on a number of self-report measures. In general, however, the relevant measures (actual acts of violence) for such a population have been difficult to validate. For this reason an experimental study has been designed in which a variety of measures are being used which estimate the skills learned in treatment and is in the first phase of being carried out. Moreover, new instruments, such as a behavior role play test, are being developed which are linked to several of the hypotheses.

The major hypothesis of this study (Rose, 1986) is that the multimethod group program will result in a greater decrease in violent behavior, and increase in adaptive responses to stressful situations than the nondirective self-help groups. In order to test this hypothesis, subjects are to be recruited from men referred to programs for the prevention of abuse to women at several diffent agencies throughout the country. These men will be interviewed and placed in an Orientation group for two to four weeks (one or two hourly sessions).

When sufficient numbers are recruited, the men will be randomly assigned to one of the two experimental conditions and one of two groups in each condition. They will be tested again following the twelve week program and once again six months after the termination of treatment. The group leaders will be experts in the given procedure to be used. (They are now being or have already been trained.) The dependent measures are a stress situation simulation test, attitudinal inventories, violent act self and spouse report, an anger index, an assertion inventory, and the conflict tactics scale. In addition to testing the effectiveness of the multimethod group approach, in general, because of the scope of the study we shall also be able to explore who can best use each of the two programs. If the hypothesis is confirmed that the multimethod group approach is indeed more effective than the Batterers Anonymous approach, one additional piece of evidence exists to lend confidence about the broad effectiveness of multimethod group treatment and specific support for its use in the treatment of male violence.

CONCLUSION

What is the implication of this research for social work and other clinical practitioners? The major result is that group workers have available to them an empirically and clinically supported approach which can be tested in their own setting with their own clients. Although the results thus far are not overwhelming they are sufficient (with the exception of the spouse abuse program which has not yet been culminated) to use the approach at least for stress-related problems and pain management in comparison with all other specified alternatives for which no evidence as yet exists.

Each of the above projects has produced a training manual (e.g., Rose, Tallant, and Tolman, 1985, for stress; Rose and Subramanian, 1985, for pain) or makes use of one produced by others (e.g., Edleson, Miller, and Stone, 1983, for anger control). These manuals are available to practitioners on request from the authors. They contain the exercises, agendas, mini-lectures, and forms used in the actual program. Most also have a substantial bibliography or suggested reading list for the practitioner to further amplify his or her knowledge about the program and a theoretical introduction.

The method and the measurement instruments are sufficiently explicit in the training manuals and/or detailed research reports to enable the clinical researcher either to replicate them or to apply them to another population in a somewhat modified form or to try out a data-based case study.

The multimethod group approach is by no means perfected. There remains the gigantic tasks of further refinement, discovering the crucial elements within the program, broadening the scope of the program, determining who can best use the program, determining the characteristics of effective leaders and so forth. However, a beginning has been made. The unified efforts of many in the development of a program are beginning to show results.

As the reader may have noted, the development of an empirically based program is a complex process, involving many studies over a long period of time. Nevertheless, it is clear that no one study is sufficient to either reject or support a given program. Moreover, such a developmental process is possible, as we are in the process of demonstrating, and is necessary if we are to develop an empirical foundation for our clinical efforts.

BIBLIOGRAPHY

Bandura, A. Psychotherapy based upon modeling principles. In A. Bergin & S. Garfield (Eds.), *Handbook of psychotherapy and behavior change*. New York: Wiley, 1971.

Bernstein, D. A. & Borkovec, T. D. *Progressive relaxation training: A manual for the helping professions.* Chicago, Research Press, 1973.

Cartwright, D. & Zander, A. (Eds.) *Group dynamics: Research and theory,* (3rd edition). Evanston, Illinois: Row, Peterson and Company, 1968.

Decker, T., Williams, J., & Hall, D. Preventive training in management of stress for reduction of physiological symptoms through increased cognitive and behavioral controls. *Psychological Reports,* 1982, *50,* 1327–1334.

Derogatis, L. *SCL-90-R Manual-1.* Baltimore: Johns Hopkins University Press, 1977.

Edleson, J. L. Working with men who batter. *Social Work,* 1984, *29,* 237–242.

Edleson, J. L., Miller, D. M., Stone, G. W., & Chapman. *Counseling men who batter: Group leader's handbook.* Albany, N.Y.: Men's Coalition Against Battering, 1983.

Forman, S. Stress-management training: Evaluation of effects on school psychological services. *Journal of Medical Education,* 1982, *57* (2), 91–99.

Heap, K. *Group theory for social workers.* Oxford: Pergamon, 1984.

Kanner, A. D., Coyne, J. C., Schaefer, C., & Lazarus, R. S. Comparisons of two modes of stress measurement: Daily hassles and uplifts versus major life events. *Journal of Behavioral Medicine,* 1981, *4,* 1–39.

Kelly, J., Bradlyn, A., Dubbert, P., & St. Lawrence, J. Stress management training in medical school. *Journal of Medical Education,* 1982, *57*(2), 91–99.

McNair, D. M., Lorr, M., & Droppelman, L. F. *Profile of mood states.* San Diego, Ca.: Education and Industrial Testing Service, 1971.

Meichenbaum, D. *Cognitive-behavior modification: An integrative approach.* New York: Plenum Press, 1977.

Rose, S. D. Assessment in groups. *Social Work Research and Abstracts,* 1981, *17,* 29–37.

Rose, S. D. The use of data in resolving group problems. *Social Work with Groups,* 1984, *7,* 23–36.

Rose, S. D. *Cognitive-Behavioral vs Batterers Anonymous Groups in the Treatment of Men who Batter—A Grant Proposal,* University of Wisconsin, Madison, 1986.

Rose, S. D. & Edleson, J. *Children and adolescents in groups: A multimethod approach.* San Francisco: Jossey-Bass Inc., 1986.

Rose, S. D. & Subramanian, K. *Leader's Guide to Pain Management,* School of Social Work, University of Wisconsin, Madison, 1985.

Rose, S. D., Tallant, S., & Lee, P. Group Versus Individual Stress Management Training, (Mimeographed), School of Social Work, University of Wisconsin, Madison, 1985.

Rose, S. D., Tolman, R., & Tallant, S. Group process in cognitive-behavioral therapy. *The Behavior Therapist,* 1985, *8*(4), 71–75.

Sarason, I., Johnson, J., Berberich, J., & Siegel, J. Helping police officers to cope with stress: A cognitive-behavioral approach. *American Journal of Community Psychology,* 1979, *7*(6), 593–603.

Saunders, D. & Hanusa, D. Cognitive-behavioral treatment for abusive husbands: The short-term effects of group therapy, Madison, Wisconsin: Family Service, 1982.

Schinke, S. & Rose, S. D. Interpersonal skill training in groups, *Journal of Counseling Psychology,* 1976, *23,* 442–448.

Subramanian, K. & Rose, S. D. A multimethod group approach for the management of chronic pain, *Social Work Research and Abstracts,* in press, 1986.

Tisdelle, D., Hansen, D., St. Lawrence, J., Kelly, J., & Brown, C. *Stress management for dental students: A multi-modal approach.* Presentation at the Association for the Advancement of Behavior Therapy, Washington, D.C., December 1983.

Tolman, R. & Rose, S. D. *The effectiveness of multi-modal stress management train-*

ing. Unpublished manuscript, School of Social Work, University of Wisconsin-Madison, 1984.

Tolman, R. & Rose, S. D. Coping with stress: A multimodal approach. *Social Work,* 1985, *30*(2), 151–158.

Toseland, R. & Rose, S. D. Evaluating social skills training for older adults in groups, *Social Work Research and Abstracts,* spring 1978, *14*(1).

Do Group Work Standards Work? Results from an Empirical Exploration

Ted Goldberg
Alice Lamont

ABSTRACT. In a school where social group work had been established for many years and where the graduate social work curriculum was organized around method sequences—the faculty voted to reorganize the curriculum, moving to a generic model. The authors began a longitudinal study of the consequences of such a change. This report of first phase findings describes the considerable differences in knowledge, skill and interest in group work found between students specializing in group work and other sequences. The findings were that curriculum makes a difference—a sequence of group work courses and field experiences did have differential impact on student learning.

The authors' interest in group work and how it would be incorporated in a new core curriculum was the stimulus for collecting data from students in each of the specializations before the change took place. The purposes of the study were: (1) to determine whether there were differences in students' perceptions, knowledge and plans associated with different specializations, and particularly whether group work students differed from others in knowledge and skill, (2) to establish a baseline of data "before" curriculum change which could be used to assess the new program's impact.

Findings are reported on pre-school experiences, perceptions of teachers, own skills, future plans and knowledge. Substantial evidence of program differences was found.

Ted Goldberg, EdD, Associate Professor and Alice Lamont, PhD, Associate Professor are members of the faculty at the School of Social Work at Wayne State University, Detroit, Michigan 48202.

This paper focuses on the question of whether standards for group work practice work. It is apparent that the search for greater agreement about what social work graduates should know and be able to do with respect to social work practice is based on the assumption that such program standards will make a difference in what graduates actually achieve. The origins of the study stem from the fact that the Wayne State University School of Social Work recently decided to develop a "Core" curriculum including unified methods courses taken by all first year M.S.W. students and second year methods courses focused on "interpersonal practice" or "practice with organizations and communities." These changes came after a long period of separate methods curricula, i.e., Social Casework (SCW), Social Group Work (SGW), Community Social Work (CSW), Generalist practice (Gen.), and Administration (Admin.). In one sense, our School was late in moving in this direction since the proportion of schools with separate group work sequences had dropped from 76% in 1963 to 47% in 1970 and only nine schools had such sequences in 1981 (Rubin, 1982). The recently adopted C.S.W.E. Curriculum Policy Statement mandating "Core" curricula and "Advanced Concentrations" seems likely to accentuate such trends and the most recent *Statistics on Social Work Education* (Rubin, 1983) no longer reports the number of schools with group work sequences.

Like many social work educators, our question about such developments is how learning about the social work methods will fare in the transition to new curricular structures. In particular, what happens to knowledge about and skill in practice with groups as the approach to teaching about practice shifts so that few students are exposed to two year programs in social group work methods? The trends have led some to have heightened expectations that students will be exposed more fully to the breadth of social work practice, will be more likely to respond to client needs and problems, and less likely to "fit" their client situations into the methods about which they happen to be knowledgeable. Others have expressed fears about the loss of depth in understanding of and skill in practice with specific modalities. Gitterman (1981), among others, has expressed this concern. Logically, it seems probable that shifts in curriculum should lead to shifts in student

achievements. If some things are added to and others sub-
tracted from a curriculum or if the elements are combined in
different ways, there should be shifts in student outcomes.
Debates about the gains and losses and about what is the
"best" curricular organization in today's world are rarely accompanied by empirical evidence to justify the shifts or to
monitor their consequences over time.

Since the authors have a special interest in social work practice with groups and were familiar with the debates about recent curriculum trends in social work education, the School's
decision to modify its curricular structure offered an opportu-
nity to study the consequences of such changes. The data to be
reported come from the first phase of a longitudinal study of
curriculum change in one school of social work. First phase
data were gathered in April 1983 prior to the introduction of
the new curricular structure. Data will also be gathered in two
subsequent years of program change.

The data were collected in a five page questionnaire which
was distributed in student mailboxes and by a knowledge test
of familiarity with the group work practice literature[1] that was
administered in methods classes during the following week.
All of the first year and most of the second year M.S.W.
students were included in the sample and response rates were
generally quite good as can be seen in Table 1. Sixty-seven
percent of the students completed the questionnaires and
94% completed the knowledge tests. All of the curricular
sub-groups are adequately represented with the exception of
Admin. majors, only 33% of whom (four of 12) completed
the questionnaires. The higher percentages of first than second year students completing the questionnaires (78% vs.
59%) is thought to result from the fact that second year students were busy with preparations for graduation and seeking
jobs.

Two further points about the study design should be noted.
The study's principal question was whether students who spe-
cialized in the social group work sequence differed from their

---

[1]The test consisted of a column of 14 group work text titles utilized in methods
classes and a parallel column of authors in a different order. Students were to match
the authors with their titles. Our thanks to Dr. Joseph P. Hourihan who has utilized a
similar method to test his case work classes for many years. Copies of the instruments
are available from the authors.

TABLE 1

SAMPLE AND RESPONDENT CHARACTERISTICS

Year/ Sequence	Composition of the Sample	Q'aires Completed		Tests Completed	
	N	N	%	N	%
First Year					
SCW	34	25	74	32	94
SGW	13	12	92	13	100
CSW	3	2	67	2	67
Sub-Totals	50	39	78	47	94
Second Year					
SCW	27	16	59	27	100
SGW	29	18	62	26	90
CSW	12	9	75	11	92
Gen.	20	12	60	17	85
Admin.	12	4	33	11	92
Sub-Totals	100	59	59	92	92
Totals	150	101[a]	67	141	94

[a]Three questionnaires were returned without code numbers and are not included in this analysis.

counterparts specializing in other methods in their practice interests, perceived skill levels, or familiarity with the group work practice literature. Two other questions had to be answered before addressing the principal question however. One has to do with differences which might exist *prior to* enrollment in the program. Accordingly, several questions were asked in order to see whether the respondents differed in important ways prior to their enrollment in the graduate program. The second question has to do with their school experiences. Even if graduates were "similar" prior to enroll-ment, it was important to verify that their schooling experi-ences actually varied in relation to their sequence specializa-tions. So, a second set of questions was asked about their school experiences in class and field work courses.

An important methodological problem had to do with the effort to encompass the breadth of social work practice in our questions. We used seven categories to describe social work practice. The categories utilized included practice with (1) individuals, (2) families, (3) treatment groups, (4) task groups/committees, (5) neighborhood groups/organizations, and (6) planning/coordination/research. These six plus an "other" category were presented in questions about what kinds of practice experiences students had prior to enrolling in the School, in their field placements, and what kinds of practice they were interested in performing following gradua-tion. Students were asked to indicate the frequency of expe-rience in each category. The findings which follow are based on our analysis of the students' responses.

DEMOGRAPHIC AND PRE-SCHOOL EXPERIENCES

It is quite common for the outcomes of educational experi-ences to be related to student variables prior to their enroll-ment. (Feldman and Newcomb, 1969). Did group work majors differ from other students in this sample? In general the answer to this question is "no." Group work majors were similar to the other students in age levels, sex, and racial backgrounds. The mean age of the sample was 35 years, 82% were female and 88% were white. These trends for the sample as a whole were statistically similar for social group work students. Minority students were slightly under-represented (See Rubin, 1983, p. 74), although in other respects this sample was comparable to W.S.U. students in recent years.

In addition to data on background characteristics, respondents were asked about the amount of social work/human service experience they had prior to enrollment and the types of tasks/activities that they had undertaken. As would be expected in view of their age levels, the large majority did have human service work experiences and, of those who did, better than 50% had worked for three or more years. First year group work majors had about the same amount of prior work experience as the sample as a whole—55% vs. 58% had worked three or more years. Second year group work majors were the most experienced sequence sub-group—75% of them having more than three years experience in contrast with 59% for the second year sample. The frequency with which the six tasks were undertaken in pre-employment experiences was also examined by sequence and the relative similarity between the SGW majors and the total sample is presented in Table 2. As is obvious, SGW majors' pre-school employment experiences involved tasks/activities which were substantially the same as their counterparts majoring in the other methods. The largest difference is in the area of practice with individuals where second year SGW majors were likely to have had more experience than their classmates.

Based on findings from an earlier study of W.S.U. students (Corliss et al. 1979) questions were asked about whether respondents had been recipients of social work services/therapy, whether they had found that a positive experience, and what the modality of service was. We were somewhat surprised to discover that 60% of these respondents reported having had such experiences, 90% had found it a positive experience, and 77% had experienced individual (as opposed to family, marital or group) counseling. The SGW majors were very much like the sample as a whole with 68% reporting that they had been recipients of such services, 93% reporting it as positive and 80% having individual services.

Our conclusion from this analysis is that demographic variables, comparative prior human service/social work employment experiences, and experience with therapeutic services

TABLE 2

PROPORTION OF STUDENTS HAVING "QUITE A BIT" OR MORE PRACTICE

EXPERIENCE PRIOR TO MSW ENROLLMENT

Year	Task/Activity					
	Indivi- duals %	Fami- lies %	Treat- ment Groups %	Task Groups/ Com. %	Nghbrhd. Groups/ Orgs. %	Planning/ Coordin./ Research %
First						
SGW Majors	78	24	18	28	29	18
Other studs.	71	27	23	29	29	26
Second Year						
SGW Majors	75	20	25	27	36	27
Other studs.	61	23	27	34	33	31

do not differentiate SGW majors from other students. For this sample, at least, SGW majors did not begin their social work education with substantially different characteristics or experiences than their counterparts majoring in the other method sequences.

SCHOOL EXPERIENCES

Since a long term goal of this research is to monitor the effects of changes in the School's curriculum, it was imperative to identify features of the program as it was currently experienced—prior to the implementation of the new Core curriculum. Accordingly, respondents were asked several questions related to the nature of their class and field experiences in an effort to measure their impact on students. Specifically, they were asked to indicate how frequently they engaged in several social work practice tasks in the field and the areas of practice in which their class and field instructors appeared to be most knowledgeable and experienced.

In the questionnaire, students were presented with the same list of the six practice tasks and an "other" category, described previously, and were instructed to check a quantity for each task ranging from "the most" through "none." Thus each respondent indicated how much they were experiencing practice with individuals, families, treatment groups and so on through all the modalities. There were strong trends for the students' methods concentrations to be associated with specific field experiences. To illustrate these trends, Table 3 presents the frequency with which students practiced with treatment groups in their first and second year placements. It is clear that SGW majors were far more likely to engage in this practice task than were students majoring in the other sequences. Fifty-four percent of the first and 72% of the second year group work majors indicated that they spent "quite a bit" or more time in this area and "only" four group work students (one first and three second year) report no experience with this task.

Questions concerning the areas of knowledge and expertise of class and field instructors also elicited anticipatable trends given the composition of this sample. Approximately 75% of the respondents were micro majors (SCW and SGW). It was thus not surprising that when asked to indicate in which areas of practice their teachers were most knowledgeable and experienced, more than 80% indicated micro tasks with 41% mentioning individuals, 17% families, and 23% treatment groups. Similarly, 83% of the first year and 74% of the second year field instructors were perceived as knowledgeable and experienced in these direct service practice tasks. As can be seen in Table 4, SCW students rated the direct service tasks as the ones with which their teachers were most familiar. Community majors' ratings were reversed. The apparent "spread" of teacher knowledge and experience as ranked by SGW students is deceiving since 20 mentioned individuals, 19 treatment groups and only one

TABLE 3

FIELD PRACTICE WITH TREATMENT GROUPS BY

FIRST AND SECOND YEAR SEQUENCES

Year/ Sequence	Most	Quite a bit	Some/A little	None	N
	%	%	%	%	
First					
BSW	11	28	11	50	18
SCW	3	11	46	41	37
SGW	36	18	41	5	22
CSW	13	13	0	75	8
Second					
SCW	0	13	38	50	16
SGW	33	39	11	17	18
CSW	0	22	11	67	9
Gen.	22	44	0	33	9
Admin.	0	0	0	100	2

each mentioned families, task groups, and planning/coordina-
tion/research. Thus families and task groups were third in
rank, but very small in number of responses. Responses concerning the knowledge and experience of field instructors
were similar to those for teachers in Table 4.

One further set of questions about their school experiences was presented. Students were asked to indicate which
two practice tasks were most interesting and satisfying to
them based on their field experiences at that point in time.
The trends were consistent with each major. Case work students mentioned individuals, families, treatment groups, and

TABLE 4

RANKINGS OF TEACHER KNOWLEDGE AND EXPERIENCE IN AREAS

OF SOCIAL WORK PRACTICE BY FIRST YEAR SEQUENCE

Tasks	Sequences			
	SCW	SGW	CSW	BSW
Micro				
Individuals	1	1	5[a]	1
Families	2	3[a]	5[a]	3[a]
Trt. Groups	3	2	6	3[a]
Macro				
Task Groups	4	3[a]	1[a]	6
Neigh./Orgs.	6	6	1[a]	2
Plan./Coord./ Research	5	3[a]	3	5

[a]Tied rankings

"other micro" tasks. Group work students mentioned individuals, treatment groups, and families. Community Social Work students selected practice with neighborhood groups and organizations about equally with planning/coordination/research, followed by work with task groups/committees and "other macro" tasks. Administration students mentioned task groups/committees, followed equally by neighborhood groups/organizations and planning/coordination/research. Of significance is that not one of these sequence sub-groups mentioned interest in a task "outside" of their major interest. No macro majors mentioned micro tasks or the reverse.

In summary then, seeking to explain student interest in various forms of practice, we examined (1) the pre-enrollment experiences and demographic experiences of these students without uncovering strong indications that the sequence subgroups varied in any important way and (2) found that there were clear differences associated with the various programs.

IMPACT OF GROUP WORK PROGRAM ON PERCEIVED SKILL, KNOWLEDGE, AND INTERESTS

Having demonstrated that group work students did not differ basically from their classmates *prior to* enrollment and that their school programs did differ substantially, it is time to address the study's major research question: Did the "standards" work? Three variables were utilized in an effort to answer that question—perceived skill levels, knowledge test scores, and interests in practice and in continuing education. In this section we ask whether SGW majors differed from their classmates on these measures of program outcome.

Perceived Skill Levels

Students were presented with the list of six practice tasks/ activities and asked to indicate whether they felt "more skilled," "as skilled," or "less skilled" than their peers in the performance of them. The distribution of responses to the task of practice with treatment groups is presented in Table 5. The tendency for SGW majors to view themselves as of equal or greater skill than their classmates is clear. Thirty-six per cent of the first year and forty-four per cent of the second year group work majors perceived themselves as "more skilled," than their classmates and over ninety per cent viewed themselves "as skilled" as their classmates. Only three SGW majors (two first and one second year student) rated themselves as less skilled than their peers in practice with treatment groups.

Test Scores

As noted above, the knowledge test consisted of a list of fourteen group work texts and a corresponding list of their authors in a different order. The student's tasks was to match

TABLE 5

PERCEPTIONS OF SKILL IN PRACTICE WITH TREATMENT GROUPS

BY FIRST AND SECOND YEAR METHOD SEQUENCE

	Skill Levels							
Sequence	More Skilled		As Skilled		Less Skilled		Totals	
	N	%	N	%	N	%	N	%
First Year								
BSW	6	29	8	38	7	33	21	24
SCW	2	6	21	58	13	36	36	41
SGW	8	36	12	55	2	9	22	25
CSW	3	38	3	38	2	25	8	9
Second Year								
SCW	1	7	7	47	7	47	15	28
SGW	8	44	9	50	1	6	18	34
CSW	1	13	4	50	3	38	8	15
Gen.	2	22	4	44	3	33	9	17
Admin.	0	0	1	33	2	67	3	6

author with title; the number of correct answers was the person's score. Nearly all of the sampled students (94%) completed the test. The mean score was 1.9 with a range from zero to eight correct answers. The distribution was skewed towards the lower end of the range and respondents were divided into three sub-groups: those with "High" scores (4–8 correct answers), those with "Medium" scores (2–3 correct answers), and those with "Low" scores (0-1 correct answer).

Scores were then cross-tabulated with the sequences and the distributions are reported in Table 6.

As is apparent and as might be expected, SGW majors were much more familiar than other students with this practice literature. More than half of the first year SGW majors scored "high" and only 10% scored "low." Among second year SGW majors, 37% scored "high" and only 15% scored "low." The somewhat lower scores for second year SGW ma-

TABLE 6

KNOWLEDGE TEST SCORES BY FIRST AND SECOND YEAR SEQUENCE

Year/ Sequence	Test Scores				
	High (4-8) %	Medium (2-3) %	Low (0-1) %	Totals N	Means
First Year[a]					
BSW	22	22	57	23	1.0
SCW	10	33	57	57	1.7
SGW	53	37	10	30	3.7
CSW	0	0	100	9	.1
Second Year					
SCW	15	56	37	27	1.8
SGW	37	48	15	27	3.0
CSW	0	0	100	12	.1
Gen.	0	7	93	14	.9
Admin.	10	0	90	10	.7

[a]$\chi^2 = 37.22$, 6 df, p = .0001

jors is probably the result of the fact that some of the second year students had majors other than SGW in their first year programs. An analysis of variance of differences in means scores found both first and second year distributions highly significant, statistically speaking (p < .001). Thus, utilizing this "harder" measure, we again found a strong relationship between program goals and student achievements. Test scores were also correlated with the perceptions of skill (reported in Table 5 above). Students who saw themselves as more skilled than their peers in practice with treatment groups were also more likely to have high scores on this knowledge test (X^2 = 13.6, 4 df, p < .009).

Post-M.S.W. Interests

Two questions addressed future plans—one in relation to the practice activities they were interested in carrying out on their first jobs and the other in relation to their interests in continuing education. Respondents indicated that they were most interested in practicing, in exactly descending order, with individuals, families, treatment groups, task groups/committees, neighborhood groups/organizations, and in planning/coordination/research. Half to three-fourths were "very interested" in the micro tasks and one-third to nearly one-half expressed little or no interest in the macro tasks. Responses about interest in practicing with treatment groups were cross-tabulated with first and second year sequence and these findings are presented in Table 7. Social Group Work majors were most interested in practicing with treatment groups with 81% of the first and 83% of the second year majors indicating that they were "very interested" in that modality.

In a further effort to shed light on the correlates of interest, each of these practice interests was cross-tabulated with the perceived skill levels of respondents. Would people who thought they were more skilled in a given area of practice be more likely to want to engage in it on his/her first job? The findings were uniformly consistent and in most cases statistically significant. The more perceived skill a respondent had the more likely (s)he was to indicate interest in that area of practice. The distribution of interests and perceived skill with treatment groups was highly significant as evidenced by the

TABLE 7

DEGREE OF INTEREST IN PRACTICE WITH TREATMENT

GROUPS IN FIRST JOBS BY METHOD SEQUENCES

Year/ Sequence	Very Interested	None, Little Some	Totals
		Degree of Interest	
	%	%	N
First Year[a]			
BSW	55	45	20
SCW	37	73	38
SGW	81	19	21
CSW	33	67	9
Second Year			
SCW	25	75	16
SGW	83	17	18
CSW	11	89	9
Gen.	33	67	9
Admin.	0	100	2

$a \chi^2 = 11.84$, 3 df, p = .008

findings in Table 8. Nearly 80% of those who saw themselves as being more skilled than their classmates in practice with treatment groups were interested in such practice on their first jobs in contrast with only 15% of those who rated themselves as less skilled.

A final area of interest which we thought might be subject to a longitudinal effect had to do with the continuing education interests of these and subsequent students. The question

TABLE 8

PERCEIVED SKILL IN PRACTICE WITH TREATMENT GROUPS BY

INTEREST IN SUCH PRACTICE EXPERIENCES

Interests	Perceived Skill Levels			
	More Skilled	As Skilled	Less Skilled	Totals
	%	%	%	N
Some, A				
Great Deal	78	60	15	46
None, Little	22	40	85	45

$X^2 = 19.73$, 2 df, $p = .0001$

was posed—after you have graduated (and assuming that money is not a problem) which two of the presented tasks would you be most interested in studying? Combining the two choices, the total sample's preference were to study practice with families (N = 90), individuals (N = 51), and treatment groups (N = 49). Social Group Work majors were much more likely to mention practice with treatment groups than other students with 38% (11 of 29) of the first year and 50% (10 of 20) of the second year respondents mentioning this task being SGW students. On the whole, these graduates want to continue studying the tasks at which they already feel most competent just as they expressed similar interest in practicing them in their first jobs.

Other Predictors of Program Outcomes

Our familiarity with research indicating that student attributes before school are often associated with program outcomes (Feldman and Newcomb, 1969) led to the search for similar relationships in this study. We did find evidence of effects emanating from the pre-school experiences of these students but they were not related to sequence majors. There was a statistically significant correlation between the amount of practice with treatment groups prior to school and in the students' first year field placements. (Kendall Tau was .25, N = 63, p < .02). Students who spent more time practicing with treatment groups in their first year field placements were more likely to have had such experiences in their pre-school jobs *irrespective* of sequence majors. Pre-school experiences with treatment groups were also predictive of respondent perceptions of their skill levels with this task (Kendall coefficient was .31, N = 66, p = .002). Previous experiences were not correlated with test scores nor with the future practice interests of these students. Our conclusion is that there is a tendency for pre-school experiences to predict what students *do* in the practicum at least in the first year of the graduate program. Some students with prior experiences in practice with treatment groups specialize in other method sequences, do not develop knowledge backgrounds, and are less inclined to continue with this area of practice following graduation.

DISCUSSION

Before proceeding to discuss the implications of these findings, two limitations of these data should be underscored. Our original question was whether group work standards worked. By "working" we had in mind that persons who are trained in a program with standards for group work content in place are more likely to have the knowledge and skill required for sound professional practice. We have not measured practice *competence* or *knowledge*. Instead, we tried to approach those dimensions by assessing student *perceptions* of their skill levels in practice with treatment groups and their ability to *match authors with texts* about group work. We realize that our measures only approach operationalizing the concepts in which we are most interested. Yet, the pattern of relationships which have already been reported suggests that there is a validity and reliability to the variables assessed and the methods of assessing them. While self-ratings are not the same as actual skill in practice with groups we believe the two are related and that our measure is a valid indicator of this ability and Radin's (1974) findings support the validity of this view. Similarly, matching titles with authors is not the same as knowing the literature about group work. Yet we believe that this brief knowledge test turned out to be a simple method of securing a reasonable estimate of the distribution of knowledge among these students. However, we are in no position to assure the reader that our faith is justified. With this caution in mind, the reader's attention is turned to our view about the important conclusions to be drawn from this study and the implications for curriculum building and research in the future.

CONCLUSIONS

Five conclusions seem justified from these findings.

1. There is little evidence to suggest that students majoring in the several methods curricula at the Wayne State University School of Social Work differ in substantial ways from each other prior to their enrollment in the graduate program. *Group Work majors do not seem to differ from their classmates.*
2. There is substantial evidence that *standards are in place.* Students majoring in the several method sequences have differing experiences in their first and second year field placements. They also perceive their class and field instructors as having competencies appropriate to the goals of these programs.
3. *The standards appear to work.* Group work students (as well as their counterparts in other sequences) have perceptions of their skill levels and interests in practice and further education which differentiate them from students with other majors and in expected directions. The Social Group Work majors also score significantly higher on the knowledge test focused upon group work literature. Most of these differences are statistically significant and several of the outcomes are correlated with each other.
4. While there was impressive evidence of the existence of schooling differences based upon the method sequences, there was also evidence that the *standards are not uniformly experienced by all students.* Some Social Group

Work majors (as well as students in other sequences) did not have the expected field experiences and were not exposed to faculty and field instructors with the expected knowledge and experience.

5. A final conclusion is that we did find evidence of effects emanating from the pre-school experiences of these students, but they were not related to their sequence majors. Our *conclusion is that there is a tendency for pre-school experiences to predict what students do in the practicum* at least in the first year of the graduate program.

IMPLICATIONS

Given the changes in how practice methods are taught nationally and at our School, what are the implications of these feelings? Several questions surfaced for us and we conclude the paper with a brief discussion of them.

1. If group work is a modality that is important for students to experience and learn, how can one be assured that it will be taught and experienced in sufficient measure to achieve a moderate level of competence? Our findings were that 72% of the first and 53% of the second year Social Case Work majors reported having little experience with this practice area. Similarly, 46% of the first and 28% of the second year Social Group Work majors reported having only "a little" experience in practice with treatment groups. Similar variability within the other method sequences might be noted. The point is that the current program, *even with the method specializations,* does not appear to assure that all majors will experience in the field the kinds of activities designed to produce the expected learning.

2. This leads to a second implication—will it be possible to provide in the new Core curriculum the broader range of experiences designed for *all* first year students? The paucity of such a breadth of experiences among the large majority of these students, the fact that they do not experience their class and field instructors as knowledgeable

or experienced in all areas, and the fact that most are not interested in macro practice suggest that the newer and broader goals pose significant challenges in implementation. Our assumption is that these findings are not unique to Wayne students. We are curious about the degree to which students in other schools are able to achieve standard outcomes.

3. Is there a limit to *how much* can be accomplished satisfactorily in a core program? How do we balance breadth and specificity? To what extent can *all* students be expected to learn about the breadth of social work practice? How are standards for such programs selected and operationalized?

That clear standards seem likely to have an impact on student learning is evidenced in this study by the sharp differences between students in the various sequences in their skills and interests. Even though prior experience predicted to some extent activities which students were likely to undertake in the field, it was their program majors which predicted their future interests. Students who majored in group work were most likely to be skilled in it and to plan to continue learning about and practicing it. One concludes from this that no matter how schools of social work define their Core and Advanced Concentration curricula, it will be critical for them to be as specific as possible about what the group work knowledge and skill objectives are to be. Who should be expected to become proficient in work with treatment groups? Would it be expected of *all* students electing "interpersonal" methods or their equivalents? Will standards for group work pose a constraint in movement towards other curricular goals?

The findings suggest that having experience in class and field with teachers and field instructors knowledgeable about "group work" does make a difference. The findings, however, do not yield quantitative implications—how much teaching and learning is needed for impact? Further exploration and trial will be required to determine this aspect of curriculum development.

We conclude from this study that experiencing programs with specific content and field experiences regarding social work with groups is likely to be associated with graduates who will utilize groups in their practice with some degree of knowledge and skill. Previous follow-up studies of Wayne graduates suggest that this is so. (See Johns et al. 1978 and Bamberger, et al. 1981). Our view of the challenge for the immediate future is to specify the objectives about social work with groups carefully, to monitor systematically the results of these efforts and to apply our growing understanding to the building of social work curricula.

BIBLIOGRAPHY

Bamberger, Jane; Caknipe, Doreen; Gonser, Ronald; Kobe, Patricia; Rose, Deborah; Tjhin, Emily; Urbach-Warsh, Deborah; and Grossman-Weisz, Amy. "From Graduate School to the Job Market: A Follow-Up Study of 1978 and 1979 MSW Graduates." Unpublished Master's Research Project, School of Social Work, Wayne State University, 1981.

Corliss, Judith; Fontana, Eileen; Hawkins, Deborah; Ramsey, Leola; Riley, Barbara; Shea, Wesley; Tucker, Norma; Uday, Marcey; Zigman, Jacqueline. *Factors Influencing Sequence Selection of First Year Master of Social Work Students at Wayne State University.* Unpublished Master's Research Project, School of Social Work, Wayne State University, 1979.

Feldman, Kenneth A. and Newcomb, Theodore M. *The Impact of College on Students. Volume I—An Analysis of Four Decades of Research.* San Francisco, California: Jossey-Bass, Inc., Publishers, 1969.

Gitterman, Alex. "Group Work Content in an Integrated Methods Curriculum." In *Social Work With Groups—Proceedings 1979 Symposium.* Louisville, Kentucky: Committee for the Advancement of Groups, 1981.

Johns, Carol; Johnson, Janet; Kuper, Regina; Montgomery, Mary; Pugliano, Jim; Renninger, LaDonna; and Urbanek, Deborah. "Wayne State University—Master of Social Work Graduates: Follow-Up Study of Work and Educational Experiences." Unpublished Master's Research Project, School of Social Work, Wayne State University, 1978.

Radin, Norma. "A Follow-Up Study of Social Work Graduates with Implications for Social Work Education." Unpublished Paper presented at the Annual Program Meeting of the Council on Social Work Education, Atlanta, Georgia, March, 1974.

Rubin, Allen. *Statistics on Social Work Education in the United States: 1981.* New York: Council on Social Work Education, 1982.

Rubin, Allen. *Statistics on Social Work Education in the United States: 1982.* New York: Council on Social Work Education, 1983.

Integrating Research and Practice in Social Work with Groups

Joseph D. Anderson

ABSTRACT. The gap between research and practice in social work with groups is currently large. Yet the call for accountability and the requirements for curriculum content integrating research and practice has increased. This article promotes three avenues through which to build the bridge between practice and research in social work with groups, especially among students. These are: (1) identifying the use of empirical process in all practice; (2) building instrumentation into group work practice; and (3) using single system designs for evaluating group work practice. When workers learn to operationalize interventive hypotheses, measure the outcome, process, and leadership variables involved in these hypotheses, and analyze data consistent with single system designs, a major step will be advanced toward integrating research and practice in social work with groups.

INTRODUCTION

Many authors have echoed an appeal for the practitioner as researcher in social work, or at least for greater collaboration between researchers and practitioners (Bloom and Fischer, 1982; Fischer, 1975; Geismar and Wood, 1982). The evidence suggests little progress toward forging such an alliance. This gap between research and practice appears even stronger in social work practice with groups. Investigators of group process and outcomes have detached from the real groups we serve in social work and have taken refuge in isolated environments with greater controls over experimental variables. Research in controlled non-practice groups and small-scale

---

Joseph D. Anderson, DSW, ACSW, is Professor and Chairperson of the Social Work Department, Shippensburg University, Shippensburg, PA 17257.

studies of a limited range of variables seem the most fashionable retreats. Social work practitioners, on the other hand, have persevered in their efforts to understand groups without consulting the research. Or they have summarily dismissed the bulk of empirical work on groups as irrelevant, at best, or related only tangentially to actual practice.

Recent developments both within and outside social work make it clear that practitioners and researchers can no longer afford to maintain such mutual dissociation. Several (Bloom and Fischer, 1982; Fischer, 1975; Haselkorn, 1978) have argued that the very survival of social work as a profession requires more active integration of research and all areas of practice. From outside, the call for professional accountability means that legislators, insurance companies, and service consumers are increasing their demands for information on the efficacy, safety, and cost-effectiveness of social work services. From inside the profession, the new Curriculum Policy Statement (CPS) of the Council on Social Work Education (CSWE, 1983) requires the integration of research and practice in the foundation competencies of students. This standard requires students to learn to use research to evaluate their own practice systematically.

With the current gap between research and practice perhaps more profound in social work with groups, how can we enable students to bridge this gulf in their learning? This paper suggests that we consider the use of single system designs and appropriate instrumentation in our teaching and practice of social work with groups.

Social work as a profession which works with group process is not alone in this current separation of practice and research. Parloff (1980) has lamented what he calls "an anaclitic depression" between psychotherapy and research. Kiesler (1981) finds the supposed relation of research to clinical psychology practice a myth—particularly in relation to the use of group psychotherapy. Bednar and Kaul (1979) and MacKenzie and Dies (1982) focus on the variety of professions involved in the practice of group psychotherapy and judge all of them guilty of unaccountability in their integration of practice and research.

These authors and others (Coché and Dies, 1983; Hayes, 1981; Kazdin, 1982; Nelson, 1981; and Weigel and Corazzini,

1978) promote three avenues through which to build the bridge between practice and research in work with groups. These are: (1) identifying the use of empirical process in all practice; (2) building instrumentation into group work practice; and (3) using single systems designs for evaluating group work practice.

PRACTICE AS HYPOTHESIS-TESTING

In basic attitudes, good practice and good research are really most compatible. In group psychotherapy, Bednar and Kaul (1979) submit that "the polarization of therapy-softness and research-rigorousness is artificial and does not represent a complete picture of what is required for high level clinical service" (p. 318). They suggest that effective clinical group practice and effective research require similar dispositions, attitudes and intellectual skills. Formulating research hypotheses based on theory and the understanding of the empirical literature is not unlike the operations involved in planning interventions in groups based on the theory and understanding of group process. Kiesler (1981) similarly suggests that all clinical practitioners and scientists employ identical processes in their work:

> Both start with empirical observations (systematically measured or not) from which generalities are abstracted and treatment or manipulative hypotheses are deducted, applied, and subsequently validated empirically (through systematic observations or not). Both . . . involve at their core a hypothesis-testing procedure. (pp. 213–214)

When working with groups, we first observe members' interactions within meetings and listen to their reports about transactions within their worlds outside of the group. Then, we generate conceptualizations of their behavior and its relation to group process from which we form hypotheses for intervention. When we use these interventions, we observe again to assess or evaluate their effectiveness. Thus, in practice we move from observation, to conceptualization, to intervention, to validation. This very practice, then, is a scientific event, encapsulating the application, whether systematic or not, of the empirical process to the single case of the group. It is hypothesis-testing in nature. Kiesler (1981) explains the difference between the practitioner and researcher in the use of scientific method in two areas: (1) whether the inductive-deductive logical process operates implicitly or explicitly; and (2) whether systematic or unsystematic observation occurs. He therefore argues that

> to make his/her efforts scientific, the only additional steps required of a practitioner are to explicate the client conceptualizations and to apply some form of empirical measurement so that the data base will be objective and replicable and thus in the public domain. (p. 214)

In social work practice with groups, the integration of practice with research requires more systematic use of the common empirical process through specific operationalizing of group process and outcome variables and through measuring these. The first step is to build instrumentation into our actual practice with groups.

INSTRUMENTATION IN SOCIAL
WORK WITH GROUPS

Instrumentation in group work has the potentially powerful appeal for combining research and practice with mutual benefits. In an earlier article (Anderson, 1978), I have suggested how instrumentation can serve as feedback for the worker and members on elements of group process and prevent the development of destructive processes so highly correlated with psychological injury for members of groups (Leiberman, Yalom, and Miles, 1973). Dies (1983) suggests that instrumentation used for evaluation research in groups can move practitioners from thinking only in terms of research with a "capital R" (Random, Representative, and/or Robust samples, Rigorous methodological controls, Refined statistical operations, and Resplendent computer technology) to consider its contribution for improving the quality of group treatment. Instrumentation, especially when combined with single system (or N = 1) research designs, permits the practitioner and members to study the group more intensively and empirically. This study can base decisions regarding intervention.

Instrumentation, therefore, is the use of systematic and repeated observations throughout the course of group treatment. It permits one to study and monitor the possible connections between process and outcome variables in the group experience. Earlier Pfeiffer, Heslin, and Jones (1976) and more recently MacKenzie and Dies (1982) have assessed the benefits and disadvantages of instrumentation in work with groups and have provided some useful batteries for initiating its integration with practice. The major advantages of this instrumentation are that it: (1) encourages member involvement in the group process; (2) fosters open reaction to personal feedback; (3) clarifies member's goals and facilitates contracting for new behavior; (4) increases the objectivity of measuring member change; (5) provides for comparison of individual members (especially in treatment or therapy groups) with normative groups; (6) facilitates longitudinal (before, after, follow-up) assessment of change; (7) sensitizes members and workers to the multifaceted nature of change in group process; (8) gives members a sense that their worker is committed to effective work or treatment; (9) improves communication between members and workers; (10) allows workers to focus and direct the group more effectively; (11) aids the establishment of self-reflective or processing norms for the group; and (12) provides members some cognitive frameworks for understanding their group experience and transferring learning to their life situations outside of the group (Anderson, 1984; MacKenzie and Dies, 1982; Pfeiffer, Heslin, and Jones, 1976).

The disadvantages of instrumentation include possible member and worker defensiveness to giving and receiving information and feedback, misuse of the measures, interference with "treatment" precipitated by the measures, and experience of intrusiveness on spontaneous group process. These pitfalls are most often easily prevented by following some basic guidelines. The use of instruments is legitimatized more by fully explaining their potential value to members. This explanation tends to remove the mystique surrounding measures by describing their contribution to understanding group process and outcomes. Too, the presentation and explanation can assure members that every precaution will be taken to guarantee the responsible use of the findings (MacKenzie and Dies, 1982). Instrumentation, or the systematic use of empirical measures, promises the improvements of social work practice with groups. The use of instruments also can do much in itself to narrow the gap between research and practice. As practitioners learn that data-collection procedures are not always time-consuming, inconvenient and intrusive for work with groups and actually contribute to efficacy in providing service, their personal resistance to research (especially "capital-R" research) may diminish. In fact, they may seek researchers and the empirical literature for a source of appropriate and valid instruments. One recent resource is the CORE Battery, an outcome evaluation kit developed by the Research Committee of the American Group Psychotherapy Association (MacKenzie and Dies, 1982). This battery meets the major criteria for selecting and using suitable change-measures or outcome packages for instrumentation with groups. It includes multiple measures; elicits both objective and subjective viewpoints and evaluates subjective impressions as compared with behavioral observations; combines individualized and standardized measurements; assesses various areas of members' functioning, e.g., self-esteem, interpersonal, and social role; measures from various sources of information, including worker, group member, and significant others; and represents instruments which strike a reasonable compromise between comprehensiveness and realistic time demands.

SINGLE SYSTEMS DESIGNS
IN SOCIAL WORK WITH GROUPS

Outcomes

The use of such a package, or parts of such a package, and other specific outcome measures can lead to simple pre/post single-system design studies. For instance, one of the instruments in the CORE Battery is the Self-Report Sympton Inventory. This checklist is a standardized instrument with extensive norms and broad empirical support (Derogatis, 1977) which can be used to investigate outcomes in treatment or therapy groups. It is an instrument that members can readily complete on their own time and that the worker can easily score. Because the test is brief and has obvious face validity, group members are usually quite willing to take it. The inventory's use in pre-testing serves as an initial assessment which obviously extends in post-testing to evaluation. Because it is standardized, workers can assess members against normative standards. This strength is a major shortcoming, though, for tapping individualized change goals. This disadvantage can be countered by incorporating a "target-goals" index into the pre- and post-testing. The target-goals approach, also part of the CORE Battery (MacKenzie and Dies, 1982), requires members to identify specific and personal change goals which can be quantified and evaluated in terms of their achievements in the group process (Coché, 1983). Again, the target-goals instrument is highly compatible with routine clinical practice with groups in social work and readily acceptable to group members.

If the worker were to use these two simple measures in a simple pre/post-test design with his or her group, some important steps would be taken toward integrating practice and research. The nature of group member outcomes would be clarified without much investment of time and resources. While more empirical and accountable in the practice, the worker would have encouraged group members to establish concrete goals for change and provided a common denominator for the worker and members to communicate about the change process. Thus the pre-test sensitization contamination to small group "capital-R" research becomes a distinct advantage as part of the contract for the group work in the clinical setting (Dies, 1978). Whenever social workers decide to incorporate research tools into their practice, the instrumentation must be an essential component of the contract with members. It will serve to some degree to structure aspects of the work.

This simple pre/post design can be refined through the use of additional outcome measures. This refinement requires the careful selection of only a few relevant measures. The selection depends upon what is to be measured, the validity and reliability of available instruments, possible variations in data-collection strategies, and alternative approaches to instrumentation (Weigel and Corazzini, 1978). These decisions require homework on the part of the practitioner in conceptualizing and operationalizing group process and outcome variables and on discovering the potential instruments in the empirical literature.

For instance, appropriate measures depend upon whether the worker and members wish to focus upon particular symptoms, attitudes toward self, or specific areas of interpersonal or social functioning. Within time or resource limitations, workers may need to adopt different strategies with different groups. In one setting with one kind of group, the focus may be on remediating symptoms; in another, on functioning in particular social roles or targeting specific community action. Ideally, in much of the social work practice with groups the targets are both some personal and social change and workers will use multiple measures to assess outcomes in the same group.

Pre/post designs, even refined with appropriate and multiple outcome measures, have limited usefulness. While they may demonstrate the general efficacy of the group in practice and can aid contracting, they do not link outcome to process, or account for member's experiences within the meetings. For social work, this limitation is particularly serious, as our mainstream approaches for work with groups are based on hypotheses that focus upon group process. Social work with groups is *through* group process. A preliminary step in practice to link outcome with process is to administer change measures throughout the group experience rather than in simple pre/post designs. This repeated assessment can be based on the same instruments, be easily administered, support replications, help keep members task-oriented, provide data for regular monitoring of group process and each member's progress, and permit changes in our interventions more appropriate to the group member's current needs.

One problem in both pre/post and repeated measures single systems designs is that the small-scale nature of the research makes it difficult to determine the significance of change on the various empirical measures. In most cases, scores will reflect individualized patterns of outcome: some scores will show improvement; others, no change; and still others, apparent deterioration. There are some statistical packages available for testing the level of significance of changes with small sample sizes (Kazdin, 1982). At the least, data-collection procedures can be planned to permit more reliable assessment of outcomes. However, much of the interpretation of findings rely on "eye-balling" charted data and *clinical* interpretation. The worker may often need to use clinical judgment, here more empirically based via instrumentation, to consider the constellation of results. The weight of relative number and the magnitude of changes in a clear, positive, predicted direction needs to be considered against those suggesting negative change or less clearly interpretable. The magnitude of the difference between pre- and post-test scores required for statistical reliability depends upon such variables as the particular outcome measure used, the test reliability of the instruments, and the testing procedures themselves. In place of the ability to use statistical tests of significance, practitioners need to look at other ways to determine the meaning of change in outcomes. Similar scores on several measures of the same outcome are more significant. So, too, is a consistent pattern across the various measures used or in very high change scores. If both the worker and member agree on the nature of the results, and especially if a significant other (such as a family member) outside of the group concurs, then confidence in the significance of change can increase even more. Finally, more trust can be vested in identified change scores when those obtained on individualized outcome measures (such as "target goals") are corroborated by corresponding changes on standardized instruments.

Process

In addition to repeated outcome measures in single system design research by practitioners, process measures and leadership measures can be used. When a few selected process measures and leadership measures are added, the goals of integrating process and outcome, using instrumentation to enable group process, and deriving an empirical base for future group practice are all more effectively achieved. At a simple level, the practitioner can use a critical-incident approach and/or a scale based on change mechanisms in groups, both of which require a few minutes of each members time after each meeting (Lieberman, Yalom, and Miles, 1973; Lieberman and Borman, 1979; Lieberman, 1983; and MacKenzie, 1983). This instrumentation frequently reveals disclosures that members have held back during the meetings and gives significant interventive leads to the practitioner.

As workers find these instruments useful they may want to build more systematic and readily scorable group process measures into their work with groups. Some are available that are high in face validity, easily scored, assessing key dimensions of group process, perceived as most relevant for members, and useful for intervention. These include the Group Climate Questionnaire (GCQ) which measures stages of group development (MacKenzie, 1983), the Feelings About the Group Scale, which measures cohesiveness (Lieberman, Yalom, and Miles, 1973), and the Group Norms Checklist (Bond, 1983). Dies (1983) has demonstrated how these instruments can enhance group process and the achievement of individual member's outcomes. The efficacy comes especially from providing the data to members for their discusssion and decision-making during the group process. Another variation is to have member themselves construct instruments and complete measurements for such evolving group themes as member/leader role expectations, group norms, self-disclosure, and interpersonal feedback. When empirical measures are used in this way to assess group process, they tend to be viewed as a vital component of the group by workers and members rather than as an unwanted external intrusion.

One great value of this process instrumentation is its use in preventing casualties of the group experience. Research indicates that members are more aware than group leaders of those group members who are likely to have a detrimental group experience (Lieberman, Yalom, and Miles, 1973). When these members are identified early through self-reports and other member data, the worker's capacity for preventing casualties increase. The proper use of these measures can compensate for possible worker insensitivity. This identification of potential casualties before they occur may be the most pressing need for a stronger working alliance between social work practitioners with groups and researchers and the integration of research with practice through the use of instrumentation and single systems designs.

Leadership

Group leadership measures are a final component of instrumentation which can enhance the integration of practice and research in single systems designs with practice groups. Social work practitioners can use a variety of instruments to gather data on how they are perceived by group members. Bolman (1971), Lieberman, Yalom, and Miles (1973), and Lundgren (1971) have all used leadership measures that reflect significant dimensions, such as conceptual input, conditionality, openness, caring, and activity level. Others introduce more specifically focused scales, such as self-disclosure (Dies, Mallet, and Johnson, 1979), helpfulness (Donovan, Bennett, and McElroy, 1979), or amount of influence (Peters, 1973).

Workers using these scales can obtain feedback for correcting faculty assumptions about their leadership style. For many workers this information may furnish self-supervision. The instruments can be readily modified, for instance, to focus on those areas the worker feels most in need of self-reflection and professional development. When these data are accumulated throughout the group process, rather than simply in a pre/post design, the practitioner can gain valuable insight into perceptions of the leadership role during the stages of group development (Anderson, 1984). Replication of these studies could tie process to outcomes with leadership functions and roles as an intervening variable. These findings would add greatly to our empirical base for group practice.

The practical advantages of using leadership instruments in a highly flexible way are many. Some of these include furnishing feedback to the worker on his or her own contributions to group process, on how members' needs and expectations during the meetings may shape their impressions of the leadership role, on how workers can modify their interventions to improve efficacy in achieving group goals, and on how future practice may improve through more empirical knowledge. However, these practical uses should not over-shadow the significance of using leadership measures to reduce the gap between research and practice in social work with groups. As social workers are taught to and learn to recognize the advantages of research tools, the potential increases for their taking an active interest in the empirical literature and in working with researchers to devise more relevant and sophisticated instruments and more refined methods for understanding accountable social work with groups.

CONCLUSIONS

Much of the teaching of group practice in social work must establish this use of instrumentation in single systems designs if we are to produce workers who can integrate research with their practice. Several basic uses of instrumentation in teaching social work with groups can do much to achieve this objective. The didactic portion of teaching can incorporate instrumentation by having students complete a variety of empirical measures on group leadership techniques (Wile, 1972), personal aspects of leadership (Dies, 1977), or interpersonal styles in groups (Schutz, 1967). The observational component could require more systematic use of particular scales for sharpening students' observational skills in groups and understanding of group process. The experiential learning can improve by having students complete measures to evaluate their own group experiences and to evaluate their own practice in the field.

The call for accountability both within and outside social work requires this integration of research and practice. The gap between research and practice in social work with groups will close through our development and teaching of practice evaluation research. This bridge is best built on understanding the empirical process in all effective practice and adding systematic observation and measurement through instrumentation and single systems designs. As we move from the "capital-R" conception of research to mining its rich vein for contributing to more effective practice, we will find students and practitioners more accepting of the research base for practice. Then, the potential increases for discovering other contributions research can make to practice and practice to research. Such a marriage in social work with groups has been needed for a long time.

REFERENCES

Anderson, J. D. (1978), Growth groups and alienation. *Group and Organizational Studies*, 3: 85–107.

Anderson, J. (1984), *Counseling Through Group Process*. New York: Springer.

Bednar, R. L. and Kaul, T. J. (1979), Experiential group research: What never happened? *Journal of Applied Behavioral Science*, 15: 311–319.

Bloom, M. and Fischer, J. (1982), *Evaluating Practice: Guidelines for the Accountable Professional.* Englewood Cliffs, N.J.

Bolman, L. (1971), Some effects of trainers on their T-groups. *Journal of Applied Behavioral Science,* 7: 309–325.

Bond, G. R. (1983), Norm regulation in therapy groups. In *Advances in Group Psychotherapy: Integrating Research and Practice.* Ed., R. R. Dies and K. R. MacKenzie. New York: International Universities Press.

Coché, E. (1983), Change measures and clinical practice in group psychotherapy. In *Advances in Group Psychotherapy: Integrating Research and Practice.* Eds. R. R. Dies and K. R. MacKenzie. New York: International Universities Press.

Council on Social Work Education (1983), *Curriculum Policy Statement for Baccalaureate and Masters Degree Programs.* New York: Council on Social Work Education.

Derogatis, L. R. (1977), *The SSL-90-R: Administration, Scoring and Procedures Manual I.* Baltimore: Clinical Psychometric Research.

Dies, R. R. (1977), Group leader self-disclosure scale. In *The 1977 Annual Handbook for Group Facilitators.* Eds. J. E. Jones and J. W. Pfeiffer. LaJolla, CA: University Associates.

Dies, R. R. (1978), The human factor of group psychotherapy research. In *Group Therapy 1978: An Overview:* Eds. L. R. Wolberg, M. L. Aronson, and A. R. Wolberg. New York: Stratton.

Dies, R. R. (1979), Group psychotherapy: Reflections on three decades of research. *Journal of Applied Behavioral Science,* 15: 361–373.

Dies, R. R. (1983) Bridging the gap between research and practice in group psychotherapy. In *Advances in Group Psychotherapy: Integrating Research and Practice.* Eds. R. R. Dies and K. R. MacKenzie. New York: International Universities Press.

Dies, R. R., Mallet, J. and Johnson, F. (1979), Openness in the coleader relationship: Its effect on process and outcome. *Small Group Behavior,* 10: 523–546.

Donovan, J. M., Bennett, M. J. and McElroy, C. M. (1979), The crisis group—an outcome study. *American Journal of Psychiatry,* 136: 906–910.

Fischer, J. (1975), *Effective Casework.* New York: McGraw-Hill.

Geismar, L. L. and Wood, K. M. (1982), Evaluating practice: Science as faith. *Social Casework,* 63: 266–271.

Haselkorn, F. (1978), Accountability in clinical practice. *Social Casework,* 59: 330–336.

Hayes, S. C. (1981), Single case experimental design and empirical clinical practice. *Journal of Consulting Clinical Psychology,* 49: 193–211.

Kazdin, A. E. (1982), *Single-Case Research Designs: Methods for Clinical and Applied Settings.* New York: Oxford University Press.

Kiesler, D. J. (1981), Empirical clinical psychology: Myth or reality? *Journal of Consulting and Clinical Psychology,* 49: 212–215.

Lieberman, M. A. (1983), Comparative analysis of change mechanisms in groups. In *Advances in Group Psychotherapy: Integrating Research and Practice.* Eds. R. R. Dies and K. R. MacKenzie. New York: International Universities Press.

Lieberman, M. A. and Borman, S. D. (1979), *Self-Help Groups for Coping with Crisis.* San Francisco: Jossey-Bass.

Lieberman, M. A., Yalom, I. D. and Miles, M. B. (1973), *Encounter Groups: First Facts.* New York: Basic Books.

Lundgren, D. C. (1971), Trainer style and patterns of group development. *Journal of Applied Behavioral Science,* 7: 689–709.

MacKenzie, K. R. (1983), The clinical applications of a group climate measure. In *Advances in Group Psychotherapy: Integrating Research and Practice.* Eds. R. R. Dies and K. R. MacKenzie. New York: International Universities Press.

MacKenzie, K. R. and Dies, R. R. (1982), *The CORE Battery: Clinical Outcome Results.* New York: American Group Psychotherapy Association.

Nelson, R. O. (1981), Realistic dependent measures for clinical use. *Journal of Consulting Clinical Psychology,* 49: 168–182.

Parloff, M. B. (1980), Psychotherapy and research: An anaclitic depression. *Psychiatry,* 43: 279–293.

Peters, D. R. (1973), Identification and personal learning in T-groups. *Human Relations,* 26: 1–21.

Pfeiffer, J. W., Heslin, R. and Jones, J. E. (1976), *Instrumentation in Human Relations Training,* 2nd Ed. LaJolla, CA: University Associates.

Schutz, W. C. (1967), *The FIRO Scales.* Palo Alto, CA: Consulting Psychologists Press.

Weigel, R. G. and Corazzini, J. G. (1978), Small group research: Suggestions for solving common methodological and design problems. *Small Group Behavior,* 9: 193–220.

Wile, D. B. (1972), Nonresearch uses of the group leadership questionnaire (GTQ-C). In *The 1972 Annual Handbook for Group Facilitators.* Eds. J. E. Jones and J. W. Pfeiffer. LaJolla, CA: University Associates.